The New Health Rules

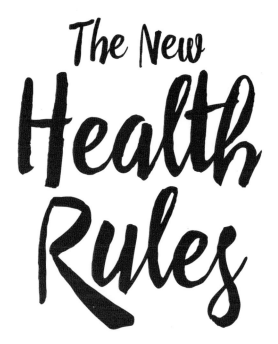

The New Health Rules

SIMPLE CHANGES TO ACHIEVE
WHOLE-BODY WELLNESS

FRANK LIPMAN, M.D.
& DANIELLE CLARO

PHOTOGRAPHS BY GENTL & HYERS

ARTISAN
NEW YORK

Copyright © 2014 by Frank Lipman, M.D., and Danielle Claro
Photographs copyright © 2014 by Gentl & Hyers

All rights reserved. No portion of this book may be reproduced—mechanically, electronically, or by any other means, including photocopying—without written permission of the publisher.

The Library of Congress has catalogued the hardcover edition as follows:

Lipman, Frank, 1954-
  The New health rules / Dr. Frank Lipman and Danielle Claro.
    pages cm
  ISBN 978-1-57965-573-0
  1. Health. 2. Self-care, Health. 3. Nutrition. I. Claro, Danielle. II. Title.
  RA776.L7675 2015
  613—dc23   2014027509

ISBN 978-1-57965-759-8 (paperback)

Artisan books are available at special discounts when purchased in bulk for premiums and sales promotions as well as for fund-raising or educational use. Special editions or book excerpts also can be created to specification. For details, contact the Special Sales Director at the address below, or send an e-mail to specialmarkets@workman.com.

Published by Artisan
A division of Workman Publishing Co., Inc.
225 Varick Street
New York, NY 10014-4381
artisanbooks.com

Artisan is a registered trademark of Workman Publishing Co., Inc.

Published simultaneously in Canada by Thomas Allen & Son, Limited

Printed in China

10 9 8 7 6 5 4 3 2 1
First paperback edition

One love
One heart
Let's get together
And feel all right.

—BOB MARLEY

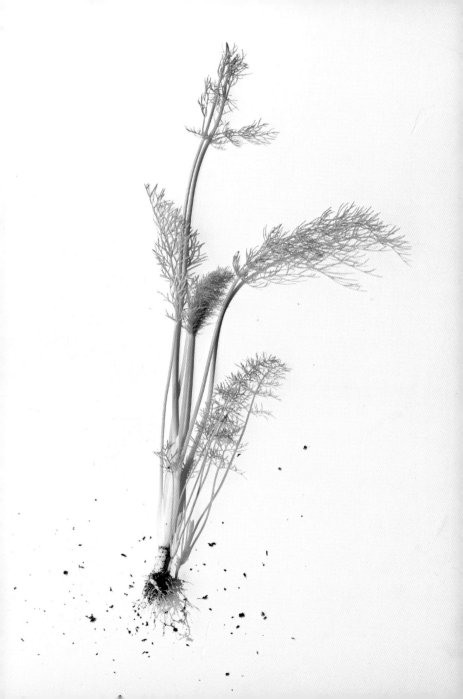

CONTENTS

YOU'VE COME TO
THE RIGHT PLACE

Welcome to *The New Health Rules*, a wellness book with a different sort of mission: to bring you the secrets of feeling your absolute best, while keeping you engaged, inspired, and awake. We won't talk your ear off or bog you down with unnecessary detail. But you'll get every bit of expert, actionable wisdom you need to transform your health. This book is not meant to change you in a weekend. It's meant to map out the healthy habits you want to integrate deeply and forever. Open to any page, anytime, and there's a step you can take toward feeling better. If you've been waiting for a clear message—been thinking, "Just tell me what to do"—this is it. Here's what to do. Change by change, you'll build a healthy lifestyle that sticks. There's no rush. Be patient, and enjoy the ride.

THE RULES WORK FOR EVERYONE

Part of the goal in taking responsibility for your health is getting to know yourself better. Not just the aches and pains, but also the peaks and triumphs. This book is for you whether you're a meat-eater or a vegan, whether you're an athlete or are just now getting inspired to commit to an exercise routine. It's about the whole self—body, mind, and spirit—and the habits and routines that make all three thrive. But it's also about the individual. Everybody's different, and getting familiar with your own specific body, mind, and spirit is just as important as the rules are. We'll help you with that.

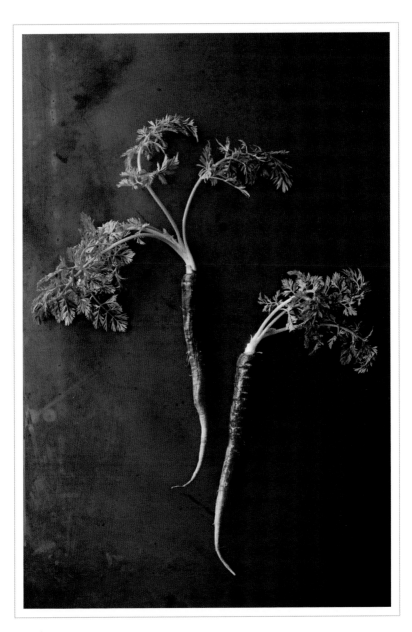

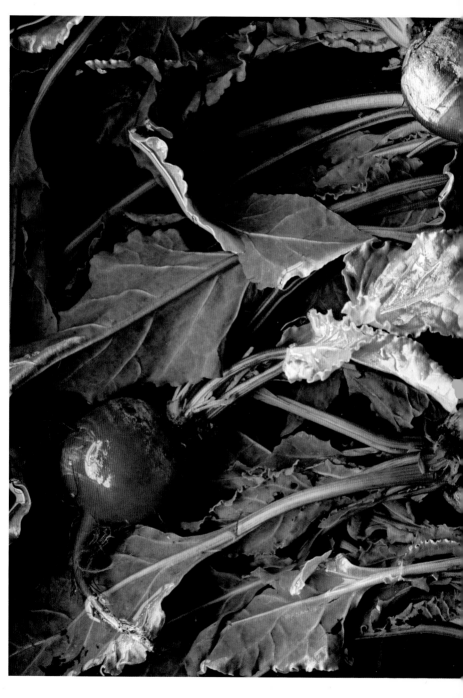

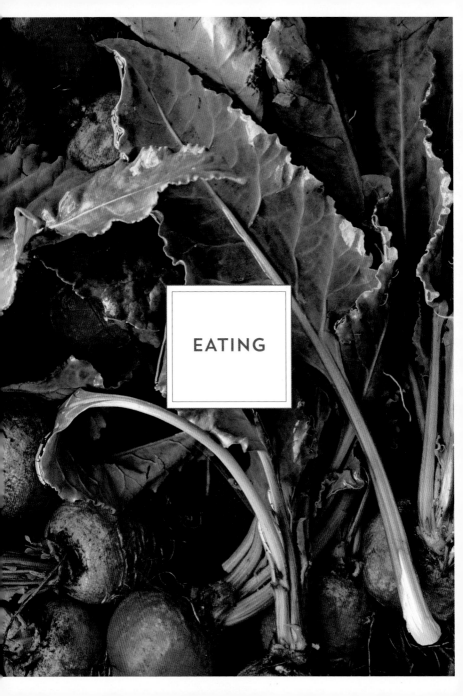

EATING

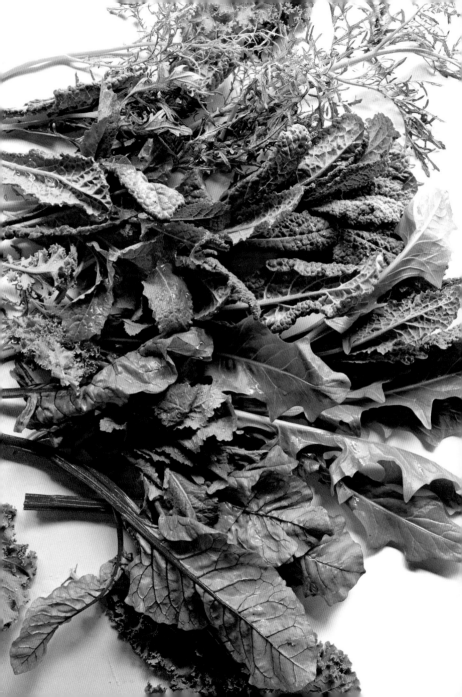

FILL THE KITCHEN WITH REAL FOOD

Meaning, the kind of stuff that grows in the ground, goes bad if not refrigerated, or has a limited shelf life. Leave no space for unhealthy items. Instead of worrying about food labels, buy fewer packaged foods. And clear your pantry of anything containing high-fructose corn syrup or artificial sweeteners, which travel under the following names: aspartame, saccharin, sucralose, Equal, NutraSweet, Splenda, and Sweet'N Low.

FAT IS GOOD
FOR YOU

Your body needs fat to flourish—good fats, which are found in nutritious foods like avocados, raw nuts, coconut oil, grass-fed meats, fatty fish, and even butter from grass-fed cows. It's the *bad* fats you have to avoid—those in fried and processed foods. Good fats are not the enemy.

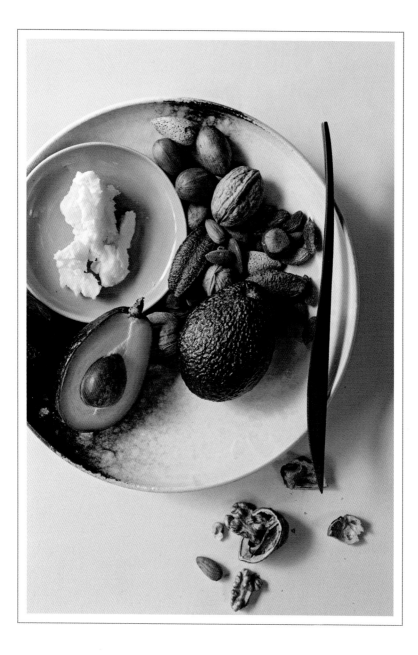

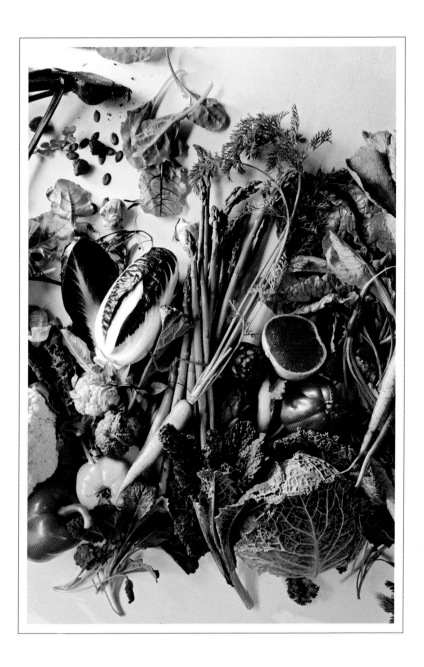

EAT THE COLORS
OF THE RAINBOW

Vegetables (and some fruits) in a wide range of deep colors should make up most of your diet. Intense color indicates loads of phytonutrients, biologically active substances that protect plants from viruses and bacteria—and offer similar benefits to humans.

BUY ORGANIC AND LOCAL

You've heard plenty about the effects of conventional farming on the environment and how buying locally grown organic produce helps right things by limiting the use of chemicals (in farming) and fuel (in transport). But this is a wellness book, and there are health reasons to opt for local and organic too: Conventional fruits and vegetables are often grown in mineral-deficient soil. They could look perfectly lovely but be nutrient poor. And the transportation process—trucking, prolonged refrigeration, treatment for longevity—further depletes them. Shop your local greenmarket whenever you can. Stick with organic options if you can afford to. And if it's possible for you to go hyperlocal (as in veggies grown in your own backyard), that's fantastic.

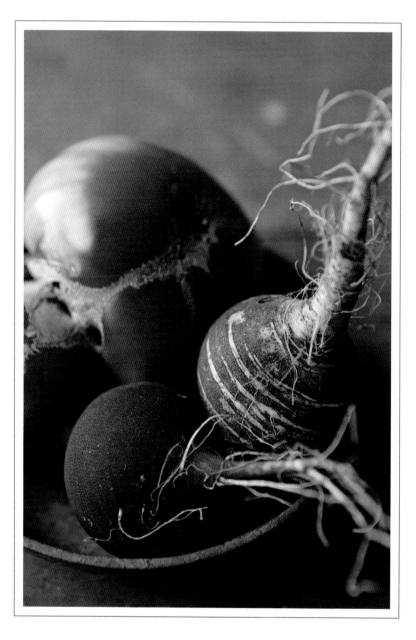

SUGAR
IS POISON

This isn't about cavities and empty calories. Sugar raises your risk of heart disease, cancer, diabetes, and Alzheimer's. If this book inspires only one change, let it be a drastic reduction in the amount of sugar you eat. It's lurking everywhere in processed food—not just in cakes and cookies, but in cereal, bread, salty snacks, and yogurt, to name a few. Raw sugar and brown sugar have a better public image but are just as problematic as the white stuff. Cut it out.

GLUTAMINE CAN HELP YOU WEAN

If you have a sweet tooth and you're making a concerted effort to get yourself off sugar, take a supplement called glutamine when you have a craving (1,000 milligrams every four to six hours as needed). It's a benign amino acid that tricks your body into thinking it's getting sugar (aka glucose). You can find it anywhere that sells high-quality vitamins and supplements.

USE STEVIA IF YOU NEED A SUGAR SUBSTITUTE

For a sweetener in your morning drink, choose stevia, a natural option that doesn't spike your blood sugar. You can get it in organic powdered or liquid form. In a pinch, you can occasionally use a drop of raw honey or maple syrup (but both are almost as bad as sugar). Don't even think about chemical substitutes like aspartame and saccharin.

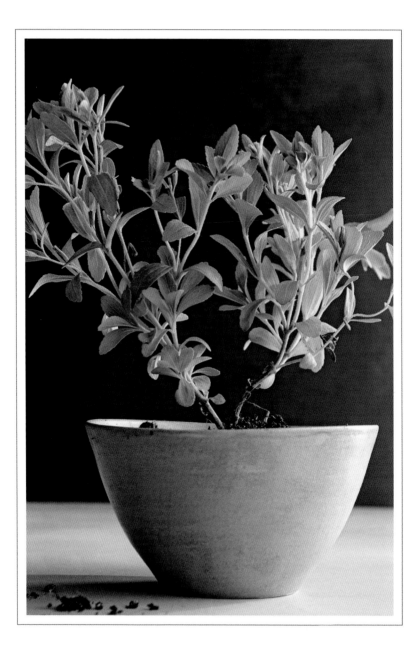

WATCH YOUR FRUIT

In many ways, sugar is sugar, whether it's white and granular or banana-shaped—and your body shouldn't have too much of it. Snacking on a nice fresh piece of organic fruit is fantastic, but don't overdo it. When you can, opt for fruits that are lower in sugar: strawberries, blackberries, raspberries, melon, grapefruit. And don't drink fruit juice: It's an intense dose of sugar—often heavily processed—without the fiber benefits of whole fruit.

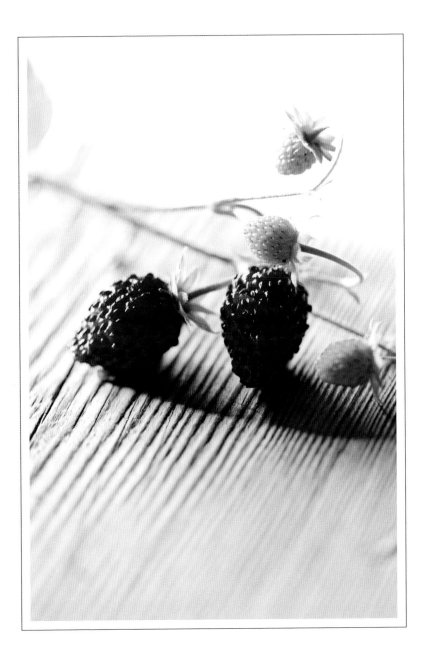

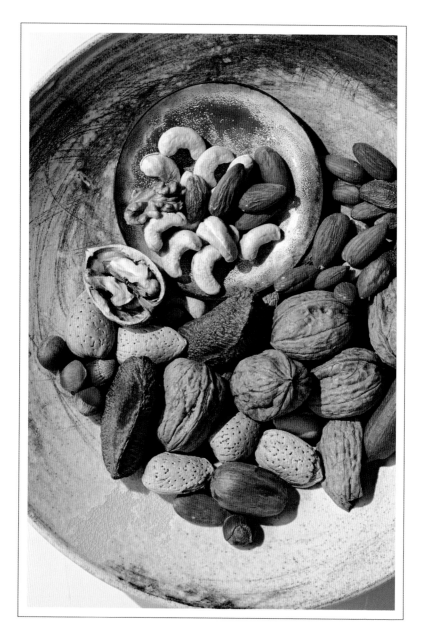

RAW NUTS ARE PACKED WITH NUTRIENTS

But store-bought roasted nuts are not. Industrial high-temperature roasting kills many of the nutrients in nuts. Buy raw and consume that way, or slow-roast at home. Just spread nuts on a cookie sheet or a piece of foil and place them in the toaster oven at 165°F for 10 to 15 minutes (keep an eye on them to make sure they don't burn). You can add a little nutritious unrefined sea salt once you take them out.

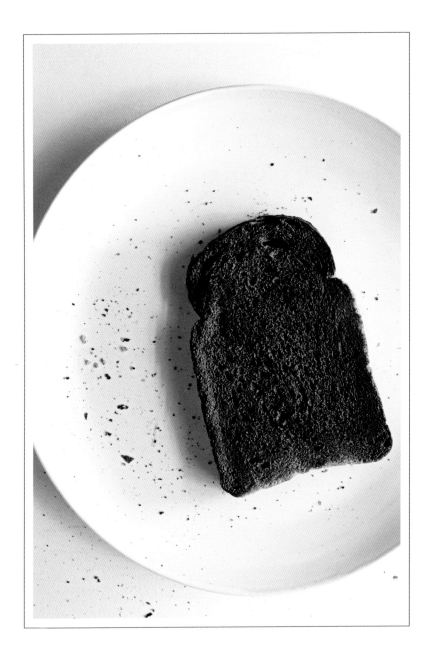

BREAK UP
WITH BREAD

Wheat is not your friend. It's addictive and an appetite stimulant, and the gluten it contains can make you sick. Pasta and bread are trouble—and whole wheat varieties are no better. It can be a big lifestyle switch to steer clear of toast in the morning, sandwiches at lunch, and pasta for dinner, but once you make it a priority, you'll see that there are plenty of delicious alternatives.

DROP GLUTEN,
FEEL BETTER

After sugar, gluten is the biggest energy drain. Most of us lack the enzyme that breaks it down, so it has the effect of making us feel vaguely (or for some people, extremely) unwell and tired. Your immune system fights it as if it's a foreign substance, and that's exhausting. Sensitivity to gluten falls along a spectrum. Most people are mildly sensitive, and some are highly sensitive. People with celiac disease, which damages the small intestine, can't tolerate gluten at all. If you have unexplained stomachaches after eating foods like bread and pasta, you're probably very sensitive to gluten (eating bread and pasta doesn't make a lot of sense anyway, since they're not nutritious). As for packaged gluten-free products, skip them—most are full of processed starches that are bad for your body in other ways.

THE TROUBLE
WITH SOY

If you eat a lot of tofu, drink a lot of soy milk, or cook up a lot of soy meat-mimicking patties, you've got to rethink things. The vast majority of soy grown in this country is genetically modified and doused with pesticides. It's a big problem. Soy can mess with your thyroid, your metabolism, and your hormones—all related to long-term debilitating conditions. People argue that soy is full of protein, but processed protein is not good protein. Besides, most modern soy products are processed in a way that reduces the nutritional value and increases the carcinogens. Fermented soy—like miso and tempeh—is better, as long as it doesn't bother your digestive system. Buy organic and GMO-free only and limit yourself to two servings a week. Edamame (soybeans in their original form) is fine. If you're a vegetarian who depends on soy for protein, favor other sources, like leafy greens, quinoa, and lentils.

THINK OF DAIRY AS A CONDIMENT

Most adults can't process cow's milk. Our digestive systems aren't meant to. So keep servings to a dollop, max. Even if cow products don't particularly trouble your stomach, they're just not good for you—they trigger inflammation, create mucus, and make seasonal allergies worse. It's a myth that radically limiting dairy leaves you calcium deficient. You can get all the calcium you need from dark green leafy vegetables like kale and spinach, without stressing your gut. And you can replace milk and cream with unsweetened organic almond milk or coconut milk. If you do eat dairy, make sure it's organic and grass-fed. Conventional milk products can contain pesticides, steroids, antibiotics, and bacteria from infected animals.

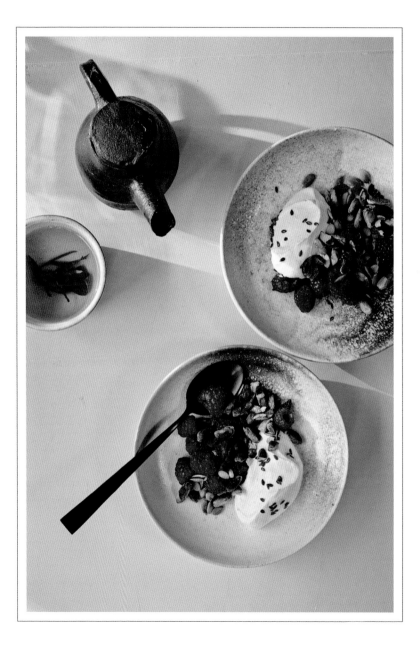

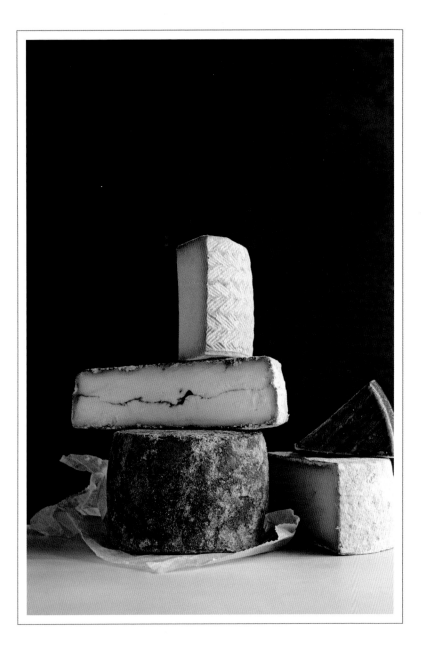

CHOOSE CHEESE THAT'S LESS BAD FOR YOU

If you feel like a cheeseless life is not worth living, at least know what's easier on your system than mainstream cow products: raw cheeses (which aren't available everywhere); cheeses made from sheep's milk, like feta, manchego, and Roquefort; goat cheeses; and buffalo mozzarella. As with any animal product, the healthier the animal, the better the product. Whenever possible, buy from local farmers whose practices you know.

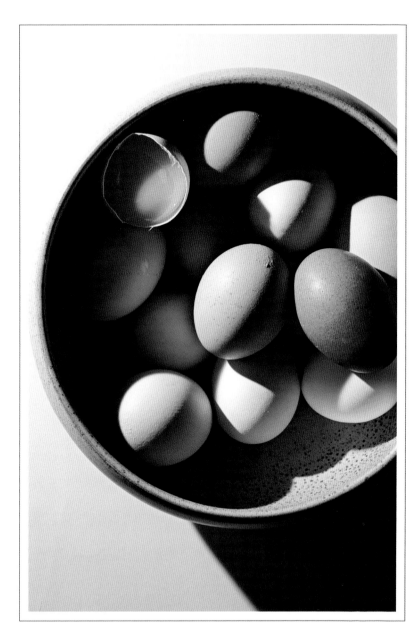

EAT THE YOLK

Contrary to popular belief, the cholesterol in the food you eat has virtually no impact on the cholesterol level of your blood. It's sugar and carbs that trigger production of bad cholesterol in your body, not, for example, eggs. So eat your eggs (as long as you don't have a food sensitivity to them) and eat them whole—no more egg-white omelets. When you eat fragmented foods, your body starts to crave the rest, and that can make you reach for something unhealthy. Egg yolks contain choline—essential for the functioning of all cells, especially brain cells—and deliver more of those good fats your body needs.

LOOK AT THE INTEGRITY OF CALORIES, NOT THE NUMBER

Counting calories is a distraction that could lead you down a path of artificial sweeteners and preservatives—the absolute worst stuff for your body. Instead, think about eating clean food, close to nature and dense with nutrients. Pay attention to the source of your calories rather than the number. (A hundred calories from kale are much better for you than a hundred calories from the vending machine.)

EAT TILL YOU'RE ONLY 80 PERCENT FULL

At home it's easy to control your portion size. At restaurants, where meals tend to be enormous (you know the places), you need to calibrate. Eat about half of what's on your plate, then pause. Do you feel satisfied? Not hungry anymore? Can you imagine a nice cup of chamomile tea instead of more food? Sit back. You're done.

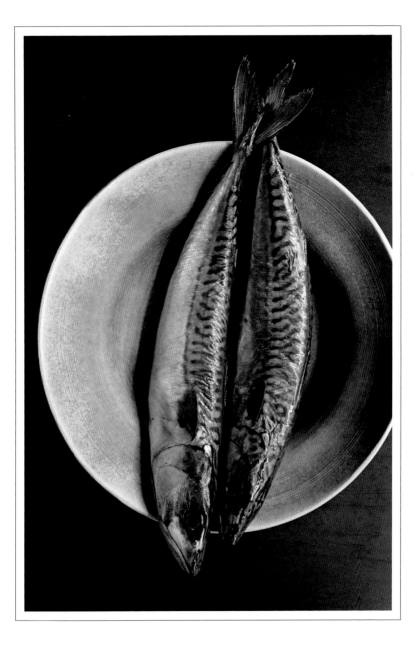

EAT SMALLISH FISH, NOT BIG FISH

The bigger and older the fish, the more mercury it's likely to contain. Why is there mercury in fish at all? Power plants that burn coal release mercury into the air, which settles in the water. Tiny plankton absorb it. The plankton are eaten by little fish. The little fish are eaten by big fish. Mercury for everyone. Stay away from really big fish like swordfish and tuna and think more along the lines of wild flounder and salmon. Mercury not only messes with your body's ability to energize cells and hold on to certain important minerals but is also linked to an increased risk of Alzheimer's. Really tiny fish, like black cod (also called sable), canned sardines, and anchovies, are lowest in mercury, so eat them freely. To find BPA-free canned fish (and fish that's also low in mercury), go to vitalchoice.com.

WHY SO MUCH TALK ABOUT WILD SALMON?

Salmon is high in good fats and protein, so it tends to get a lot of play in modern health talk. Wild salmon is much better than "farmed" salmon, because fish raised in captivity are trapped in small spaces and swimming in their own filth. To fight these disgusting conditions, farmed salmon are given antibiotics, which you end up ingesting when you eat the fish. But wait—it gets worse: The food these salmon eat is mixed with GMO soy and corn. These fish grow up gray-colored and are later dyed orangey-pink. Wild salmon, on the other hand, are naturally pink from eating shrimp—and they're antibiotic and chemical free.

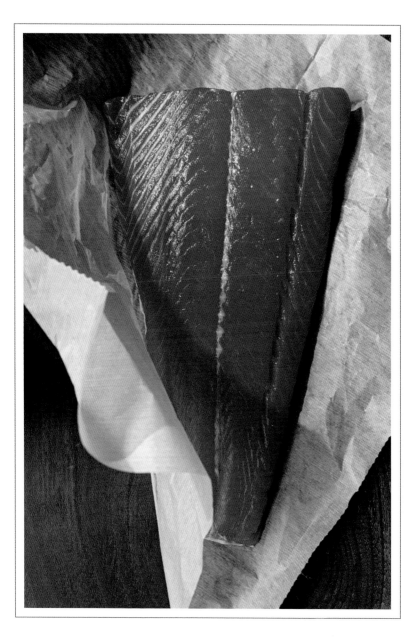

GMOS SHOULD NOT BE A PART OF YOUR DIET

Genetically modified organism refers to crops whose seeds have been altered in labs—they've been injected with substances like hormones, antibiotics, and pesticides to resist disease and drought. The stuff shot into the seeds grows into the food. And this food appears to be making people sick. Since this practice started in the United States, chronic illnesses and allergies have skyrocketed. Avoid GMOs by buying local and organic whenever possible. For help in the supermarket aisles, make sure any nonorganic packaged foods you buy have a stamp from the Non-GMO Project (go to nongmoproject.org to see the label so you can easily spot it in the store).

CAFFEINE CAN HAVE A HALF-LIFE OF SEVEN HOURS

If you're a slow metabolizer of caffeine (many people are), seven hours after you drink a cup of coffee, half the caffeine is still in your system. Which means a 4:00 P.M. Starbucks can block your sleep neurotransmitters and throw off your natural rhythms, leaving you tossing and turning at 11:00. Caffeine also excites the adrenal glands, which help regulate stress. If you're struggling with insomnia or intense stress, eliminating caffeine can make a huge difference. At the very least, cut your intake in half and never consume caffeine (that includes soda—which should be gone from your diet anyway) after 1:00 P.M.

BEVERAGE SMACKDOWN: GREEN TEA VERSUS LATTE

If you depend on a hit of caffeine in the morning, maybe it's time to lighten the load. Switching to green tea not only cuts a bunch of hard-to-digest dairy from your day but also strengthens your immune system, helping to arm you against cancer and heart disease; it may even help stave off dementia. Rich in polyphenols—botanical antioxidants—it also protects skin from the aging effects of the sun.

GREEN TEA	LATTE
CAFFEINE: about 25 milligrams	CAFFEINE: about 150 milligrams
FAT: 0	FAT: 7 grams
SUGARS: 0	SUGARS: 17 grams
CALORIES: 0	CALORIES: 190
CARBS: 0	CARBS: 18 grams
UPSHOT: a bit of energy	UPSHOT: a jolt of energy followed by a crash, a stomachache, hunger

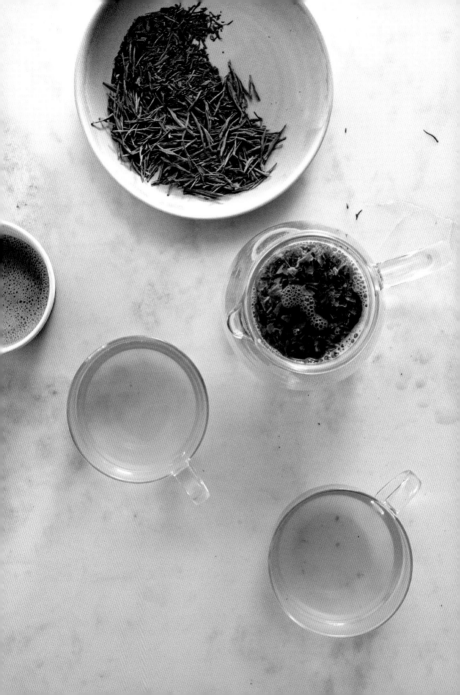

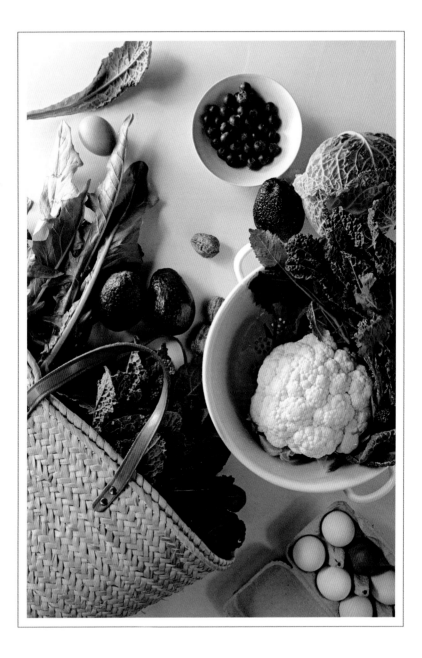

BUY THESE EVERY WEEK

DARK LEAFY GREENS
More nutritious, calorie for calorie, than
any other food

CRUCIFEROUS VEGGIES
Lower the risk of cancer

AVOCADOS
Help protect your body from heart disease,
cancer, and certain degenerative diseases

BLUEBERRIES
Help prevent cancer, diabetes, heart disease,
ulcers, and high blood pressure

EGGS
Full of protein and good fats

WALNUTS
Packed with omega-3s and other nutrients
that help protect your heart

PREP AS YOU PUT AWAY

If the good stuff is there and ready when you open your fridge, you'll eat it. If not, you're more likely to reach for processed packaged food. So after shopping at your local farmers' market or your organic grocer, devote a half hour to washing and prepping—before you even put the stuff away. Rinse carrots (peel if they're not organic) and stash in a glass container full of water to keep them snappy. Wash berries, drain them very well, and store in a dry colander so they have plenty of air around them. Hard-boil a dozen eggs. Wash and spin greens and store in a dry salad spinner or a plastic bag. It really helps your habits when everything is at hand and ready to pop onto a plate (or into your mouth).

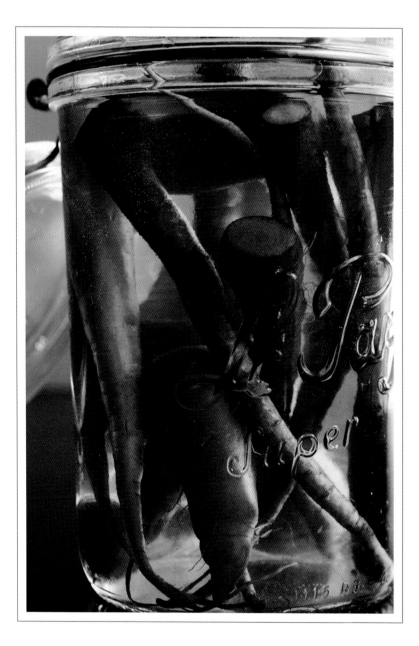

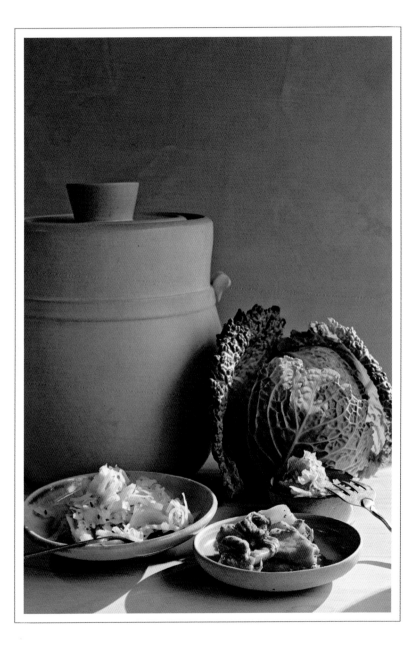

YOUR GUT LOVES FERMENTED FOODS

Sauerkraut, kimchi, kombucha, pickled veggies, and tempeh encourage the growth of good bacteria, for a healthy gut. Buy these foods from the refrigerated section of the grocery store, not from the (unrefrigerated) pickle aisle—fermented foods need to be stored cold in order for the organisms to thrive—or get a fermentation pot and make your own.

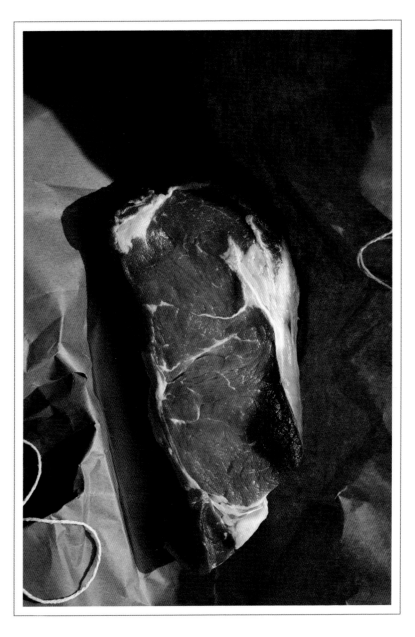

IF YOU EAT COWS, MAKE SURE THEY EAT GRASS

To save money, factory-farmed cows are fed corn (which is cheap and often genetically modified) instead of the grasses they're meant to graze on. Corn makes the cows sick, so they're given antibiotics. These meds also fatten the cows—so the system "works" from a business perspective. From a health perspective for meat-eaters, it's a disaster. If you eat factory-farmed meat, you're ingesting sick animals, plus loads of antibiotics. Buy only grass-fed meat, and whenever possible, get it at a local farmers' market from small farms.

BE CAREFUL WHERE YOU GET YOUR CHICKEN (AND EGGS)

The term *free-range* is now as meaningless as the word *natural*. And *cage-free* does not mean *crate-free* (loophole!) The best plan for consuming healthy (and ethically raised) poultry and eggs is to buy from a farmer whose practices you know, at a local market. But that's not always possible, so look for the word *organic*, which promises that the birds were not shot up with antibiotics or given feed containing animal by-products. It's not much, but it's the best term there is right now.

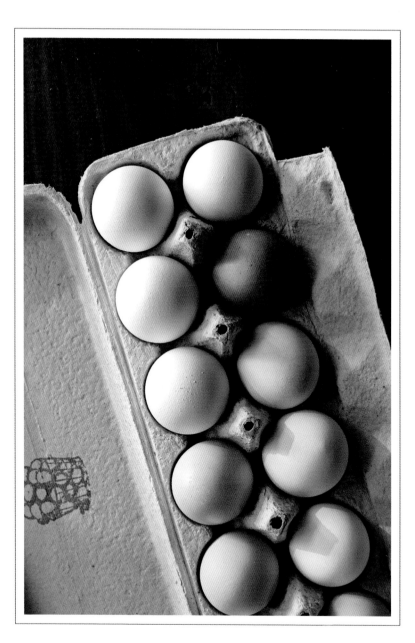

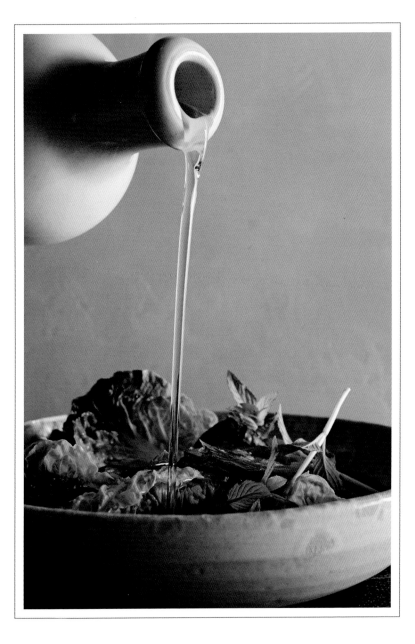

OLIVE OIL ON SALAD IS BETTER THAN OLIVE OIL IN COOKING

The good, nutritious fats you get from extra-virgin olive oil are altered when the oil is heated. That doesn't make it *bad* for you when it's used in cooking; it just takes away some of its magic properties. So go ahead and use a little of it to keep the fish from sticking to the pan. But for maximum health benefits, drizzle it on your salad or swirl it into a green juice (it adds amazing richness).

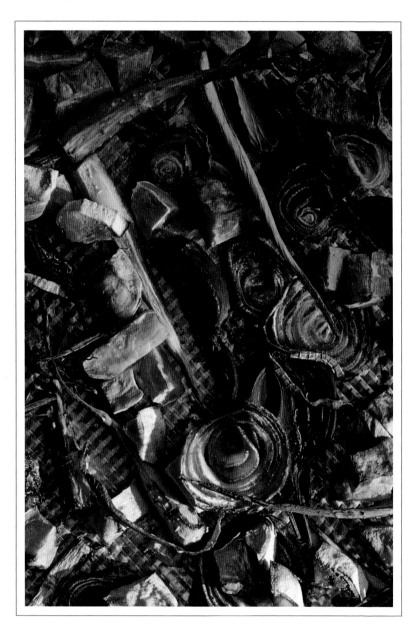

SKIP THE GRAINS; ADD MORE VEGGIES

Most of us are in the habit of having "that third thing" at dinner with our protein and vegetables—and more often than not, that's a grain. But since every bite on your plate should be packed with nutrients, and grains just don't compare, make that third item a satisfying starchy vegetable instead. Carrots and onions sautéed to bring out their sweetness, beets with balsamic, or peas with mint can taste just as indulgent and satisfying as a mound of rice. If the carb craving is overwhelming, make it a healthier carb like quinoa or amaranth (which both deliver protein), and keep portions tiny.

EAT LIKE A CAVEMAN

If you're really sensitive to carbs—and more and
more people are realizing they are—try a Paleo diet
(so named because it's probably how our ancestors
ate in the days before farming). Eat grass-fed meat,
wild-caught fish, greens, nuts, a bit of fruit—and no
other carbs—for a month and see how you feel.

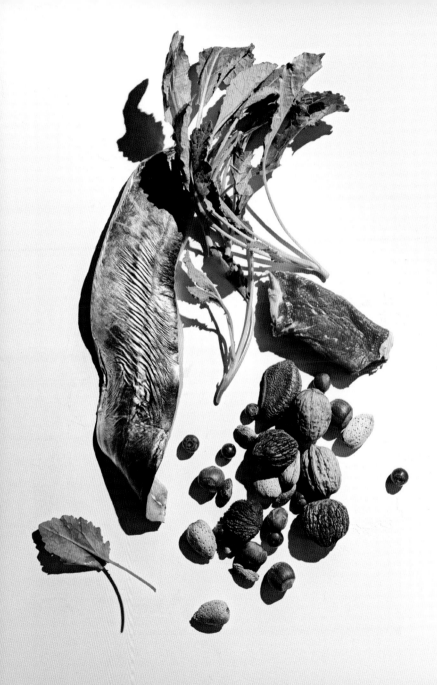

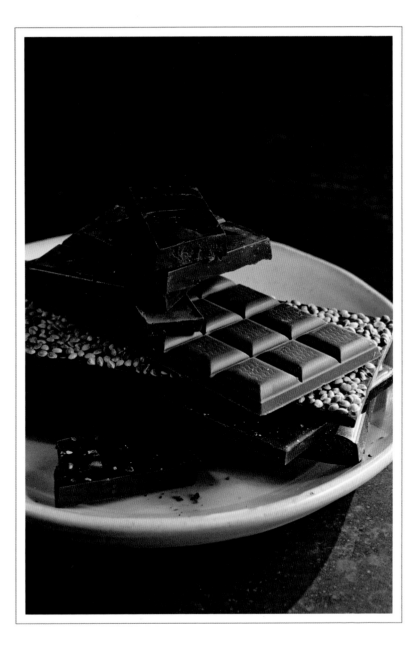

IS CHOCOLATE SERIOUSLY GOOD FOR YOU?

Only high-quality dairy-free dark chocolate has significant health benefits (improving blood flow, reducing cholesterol, and helping to prevent cell damage). Most chocolate, though, contains milk (even most dark chocolate), which blocks your body's absorption of its antioxidants. A few times a week you can treat yourself to an ounce or so of top-shelf dairy-free chocolate (check the label) that has a cacao content of 70 percent or higher. As for chocolate containing milk, cross it off your list.

UPGRADE YOUR SNACKS

The less junky food you eat, the more sensitive and subtle your taste buds become. Without the onslaught of heavily salted, artificially flavored, fatted-up foods, your mouth learns to appreciate—and crave—good fats, vegetables, and salads. So forego chips and pretzels and keep a healthful sweet-and-savory snack handy instead. A half-cup serving of this blend (which keeps nicely in an airtight container in the fridge for a couple of weeks) will satisfy any yen, sweet or savory. Just mix equal parts:

Raw almonds
Raw walnuts
Raw cashews
Raw Brazil nuts
Raw sunflower seeds
Raw pumpkin seeds
Cacao nibs

Then add a dash of chopped dates.

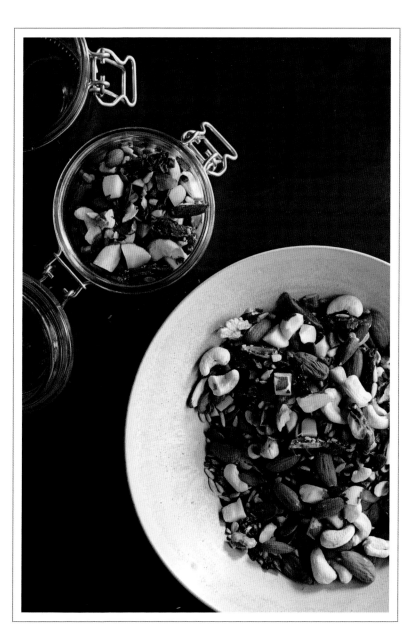

EVERYTHING YOU KNOW ABOUT BREAKFAST IS WRONG

Get away from fruit and grains in the morning—you don't need that sugar and gluten. A dose of healthy fats will start your day off right. Have boiled or poached eggs with greens, sardines on gluten-free crispbreads, or half an avocado—score it, spritz with lemon or olive oil, sprinkle with salt and cumin, and eat it like a grapefruit.

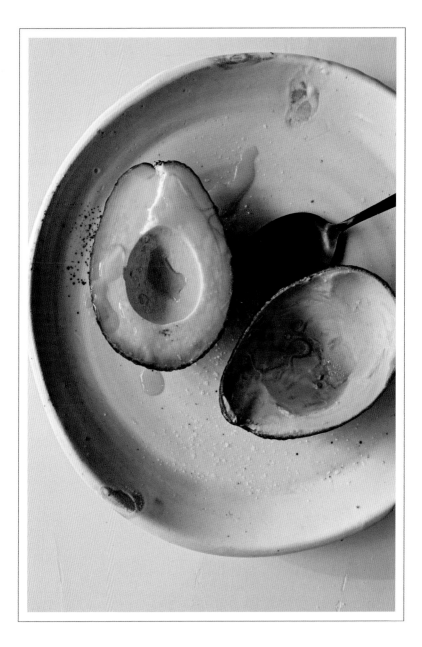

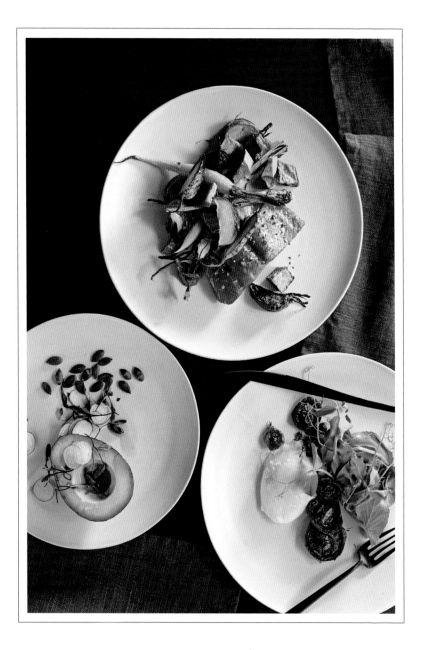

RIGHT-SIZE YOUR MEALS

Is dinner the biggest meal of your day? Time to switch that. Lunch should be the largest meal—packed with protein, good fats, and vegetables—because midday is when digestion peaks. Breakfast should be significant too. In the morning your body needs energy and your metabolism is cranking—think good fats delivered via avocado, omelet, or last night's leftovers. Dinner should be small—proteins and greens; eggs and salad actually make a perfect evening meal. And no matter what the time of day, give some thought to your portion size. Reasonable servings of power-packed foods are energizing, but a huge pile of food (even healthful food) can be like an assault on the body, overloading your system and leaving you lethargic.

BREAKFAST IN A GLASS

If you're not a big morning eater, have a tasty smoothie with protein powder and healthy fats. A favorite is this blueberry-avocado-kale shake.

4 to 6 ounces water
4 to 6 ounces unsweetened coconut milk
1 serving whey protein or pea protein powder
1 serving greens powder
½ cup frozen or fresh blueberries
¼ small avocado
1 cup kale
4 ice cubes

Blend the ingredients in a blender until smooth and creamy.

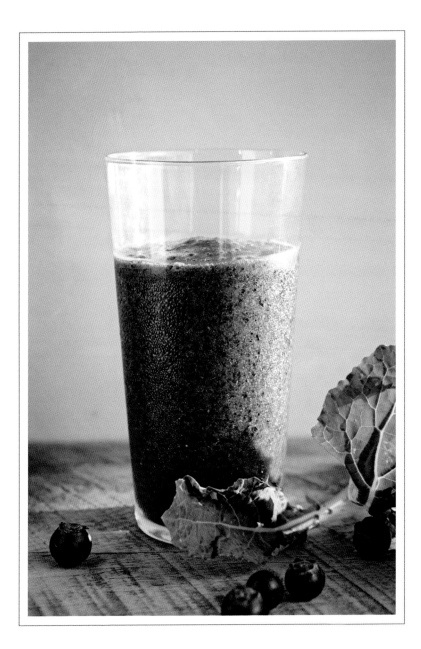

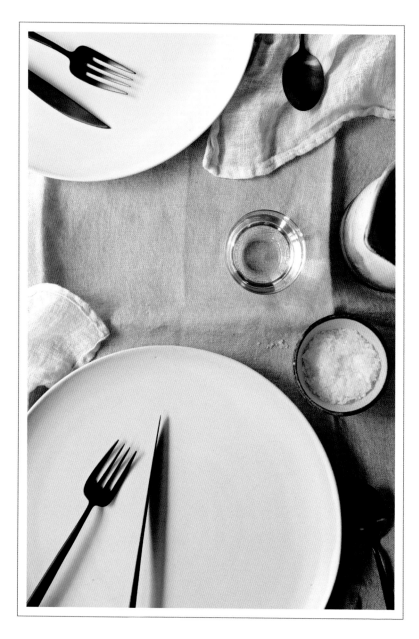

DON'T EAT OVER THE KITCHEN SINK

If you're tempted to gobble something while cleaning up from dinner, just take a minute and sit down. You'll digest better and bring more thought to what you're putting in your mouth. Likewise, try not to eat in front of the TV, and if you've brought home takeout, serve yourself a reasonable portion rather than eating out of the container. Eat consciously and you're more likely to eat just what your body needs.

PEPPERMINT TEA INSTEAD OF CANDY

To counter a sweets craving, try mint tea (it's the soothing version of brushing your teeth to redirect your taste buds). Stock some at work and at home and always travel with a few bags handy—the airport can feel like a lawless society, nutritionally speaking.

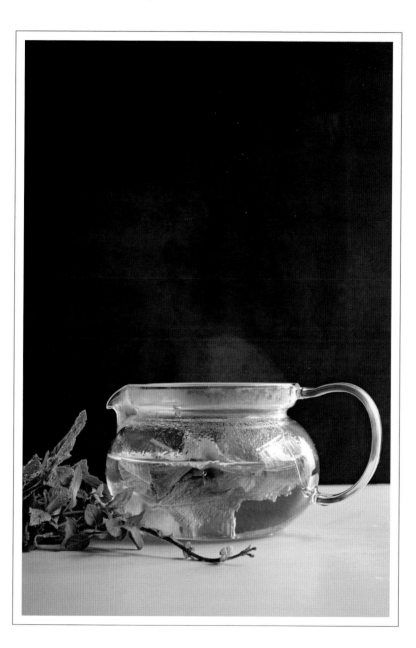

CHEW YOUR FOOD WELL

This isn't a little side note or a matter of table manners. Digestion begins in your mouth. If you gulp down big particles, the stomach and intestines have to work extra hard. Over time, the digestive system just gets exhausted. Then big particles end up in the bloodstream, where the immune system attacks them. You might experience this as a reaction (stomachaches, say) to foods you're actually totally fine with. Taking your time with each bite, of course, also gives your body a chance to know when it's full, before it takes in too much.

REST YOUR DIGESTIVE SYSTEM

You've probably heard about "intermittent fasting" as a means of losing weight. A simple, effective take on it (that won't leave you starving) is to leave 14 hours between dinner and the next day's first meal a couple of times a week. (You can have a cup of tea in the morning.) Whether or not you're trying to drop weight, this gap gives your digestive system a break and helps it work better when it's on duty. (But if you have low blood sugar or feel exhausted all the time, intermittent fasting isn't for you.)

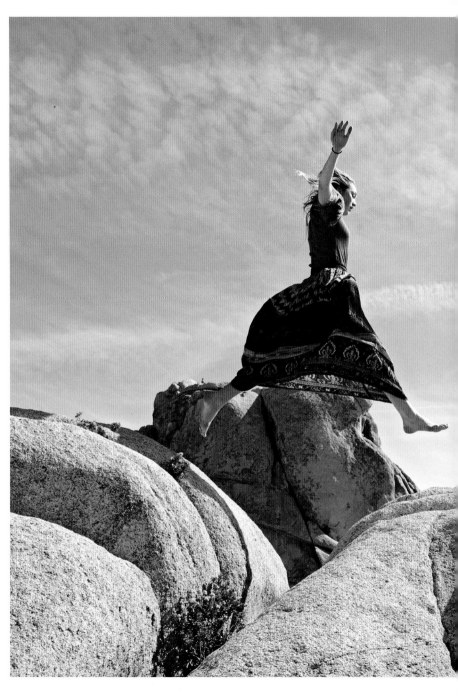

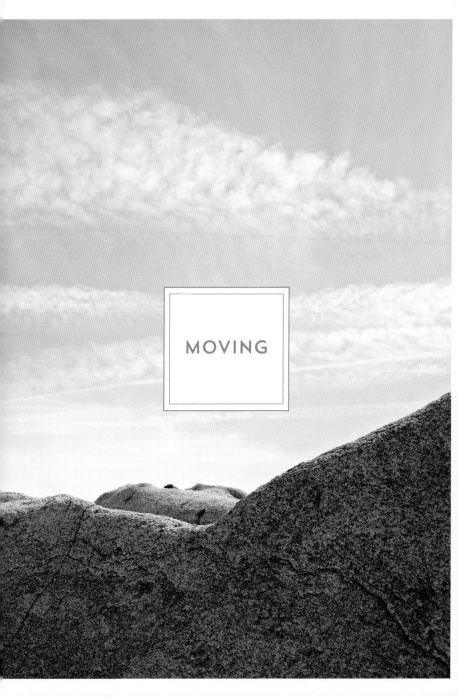

MOVING

STRONG AND STRETCHY

We tend to fall into one camp or the other when it comes to fitness—go-go power exercisers or chill yoga loyalists. Truth is, you need balance. Resistance, strength, or weight training keeps bones healthy, which becomes more and more important as you age. Deep stretching (like you get with yoga) prevents injury, counterbalances the "poses" we're stuck in all day at work, and cultivates healthy posture. So if you live mostly in column A, grab something from column B once a week, and vice versa. And regularly throw in a 10-minute stretch session after hard-core lifting at the gym, or a few bonus chaturangas in Vinyasa class. Core work is also required (no whining). It's not about your bikini belly—it's about your back. And having a strong central support for your whole musculoskeletal system. One way or another, do something physical every single day.

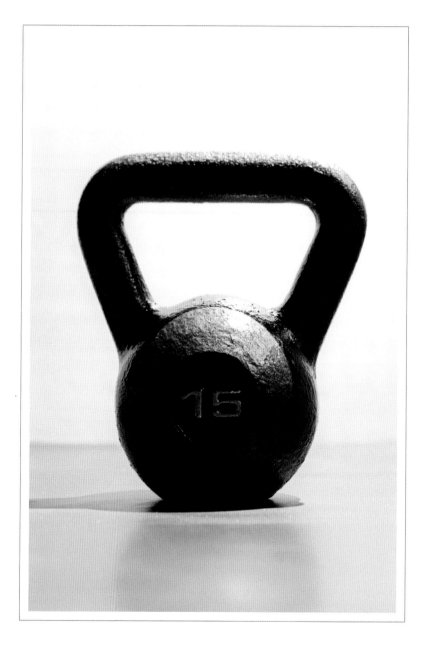

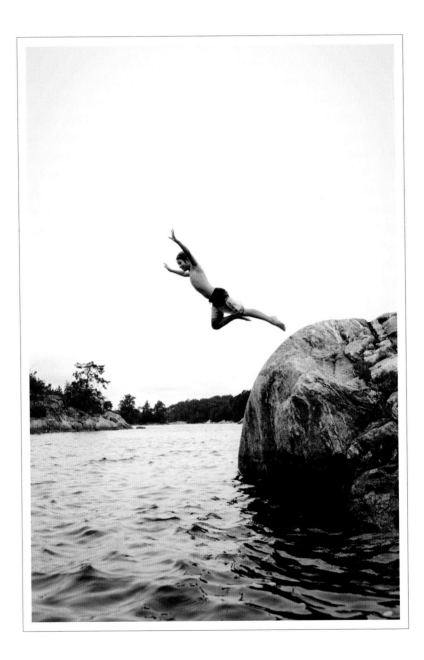

EXERCISE LIKE KIDS PLAY

Our bodies are not built to run long distances for no reason at all. We're built to chase down prey and then stop. To run from danger and then stop. That's what feels best and works best to keep us in shape—short bursts of intense exertion interspersed with periods of leisurely movement. The long-held belief that we need to elevate the heart rate with 30 minutes of sustained activity is being replaced by this plan— often referred to as interval training. You don't need a specially designed workout or a personal trainer to apply this. When you're running, sprint for a minute, then walk or trot for five. In the pool, swim one fast lap, then do three at a leisurely pace. This system is organic to many yoga classes (you practice kicking up into handstand for two minutes, then you follow up with a restorative child's pose). But with some workouts it's up to you to adjust. Worried you won't burn enough calories? With interval training, you'll actually burn more.

TRAIL VERSUS TREADMILL

When you can, walk and run outside rather than on a machine at the gym—and whenever you have the opportunity, on unpaved ground. The little bumps and hills of natural, uneven terrain activate and strengthen different muscles and challenge your balance and coordination, giving you a more thorough workout.

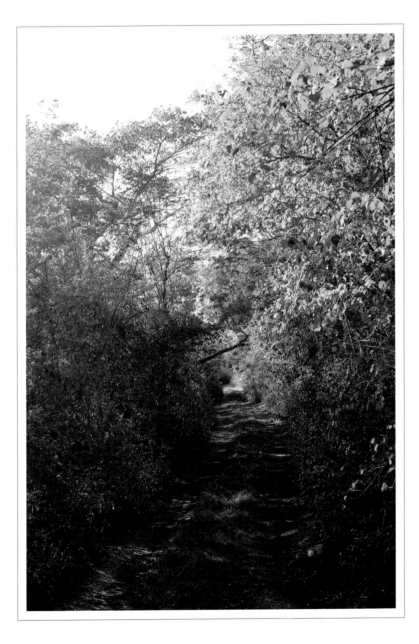

WHY YOGA IS A BIG DEAL

Yoga is about a lot of things, but largely it's about learning how to stay in an uncomfortable place. Take that anywhere you want. To your work life. To relationships. To parenting. To finances. The concept goes wherever you need it. Standing in tree pose, for example, teetering on one foot, you might say to yourself, *Hmm . . . if I shift my weight a little to the left, I think I can handle this a bit better. If I lift my chest, I might be able to breathe more fully and make this whole thing easier.* And then later, when you're in a meeting at the office that's hard to tolerate, you find yourself tapping into the same principles: tweaking your stance, finding a way to take a breath—and the situation becomes bearable. In this way, yoga changes everything. But it doesn't happen overnight. We return to the mat again and again because it takes time to embed this type of thinking. And once we get it, we lose it and start looking for it all over again. That's why it's called a practice. You never master it. You just stay on the path and keep discovering new scenery.

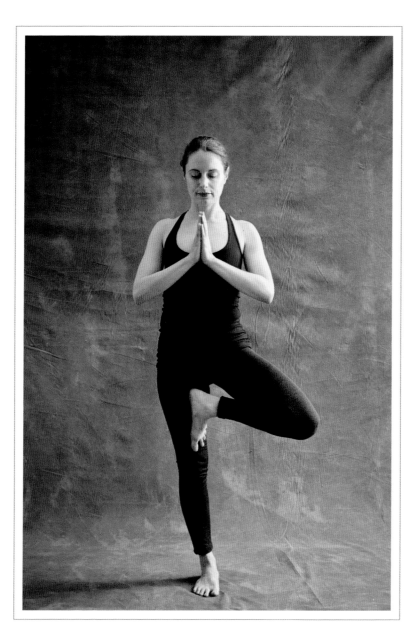

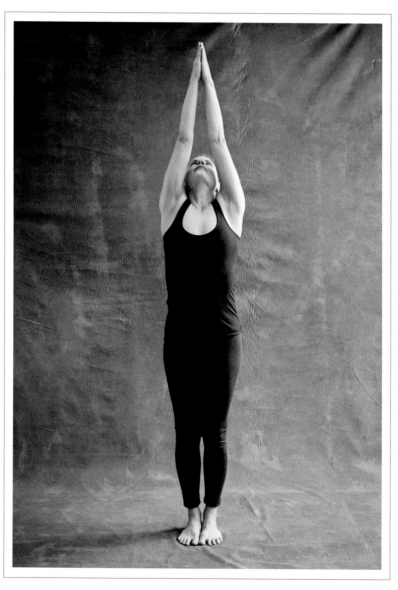

Yoga is about linking breath and movement.

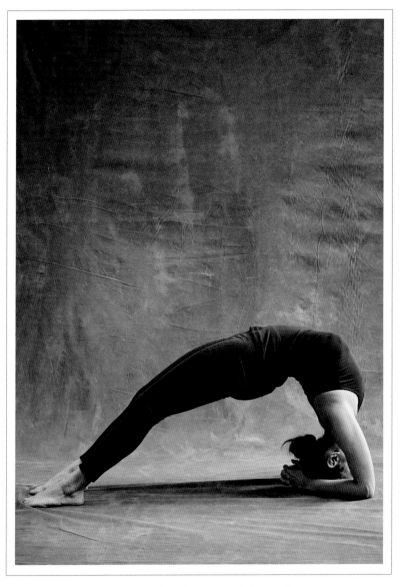

**Yoga is about noticing where your mind goes when you
ask your body to do something unfamiliar or scary.**

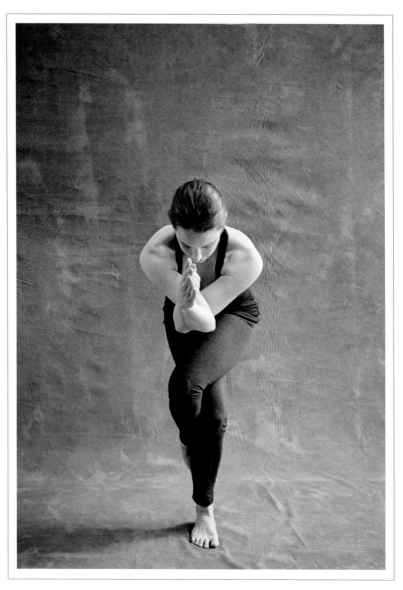

Yoga is about being humble.

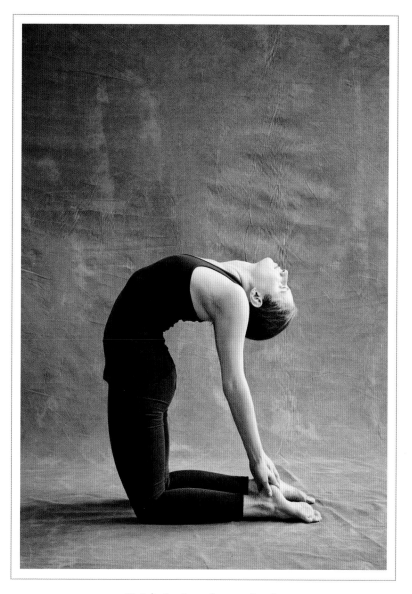

Yoga is about opening your heart.

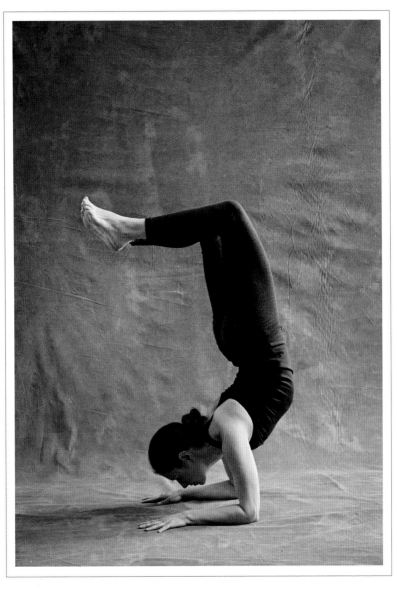

**Yoga is about discovering balance
and being nice to yourself when you fall.**

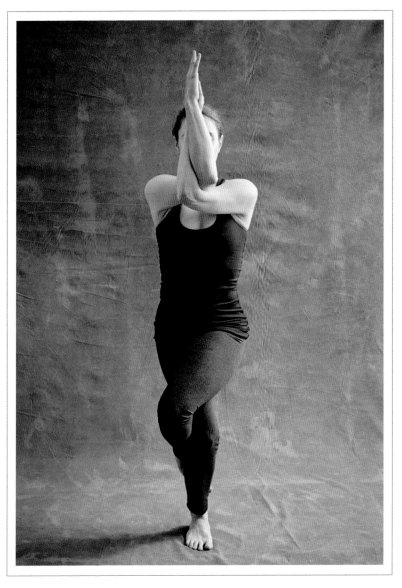

Yoga is about fixing things from the inside.

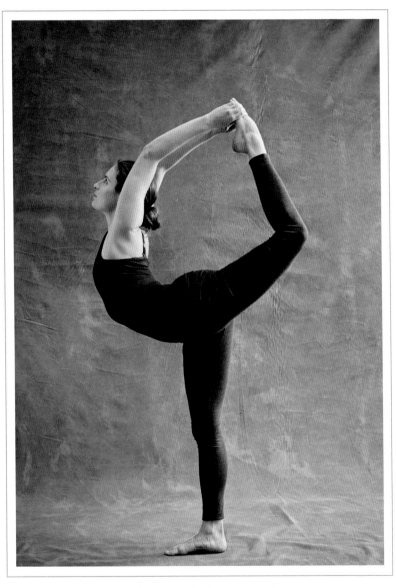

Yoga is the pursuit of outward clarity,
to help move us toward inner clarity.

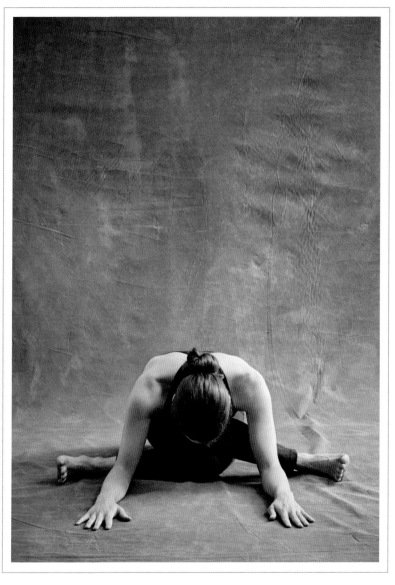

Yoga is about stretching, strengthening, stimulating, and
tuckering out every muscle in the body so you can comfortably sit
and meditate, without any aches to distract you.

IF YOU LEARN ONLY ONE YOGA POSE . . .

. . . let it be supta baddha konasana. It's a heart-opening, lung-stretching, deeply restorative posture you can do with or without props—a chance to get a sense of the magic of yoga without straining yourself. Whether you spend your days at a computer, or working with your hands, or on the floor playing with kids, you're likely to be closed and tight in the front of your body (most of us are). This helps. With a bolster under your shoulder blades, and your choice of folded blankets, firm pillows, or yoga blocks supporting knees, spine, and head, you'll feel a gentle (and gradually deepening) release in your hips, chest, shoulders, and throat. Stay for five minutes; it's an amazing way to start or end your day.

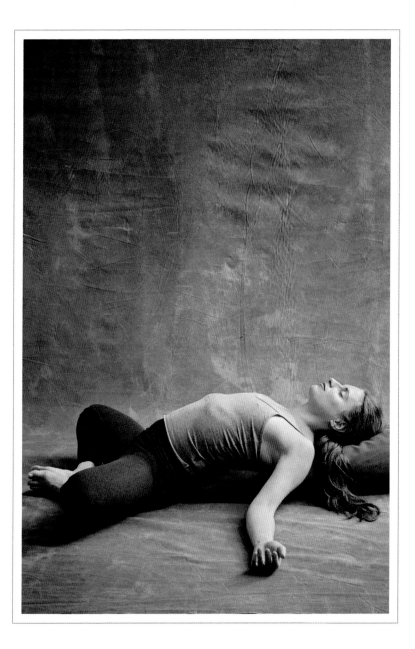

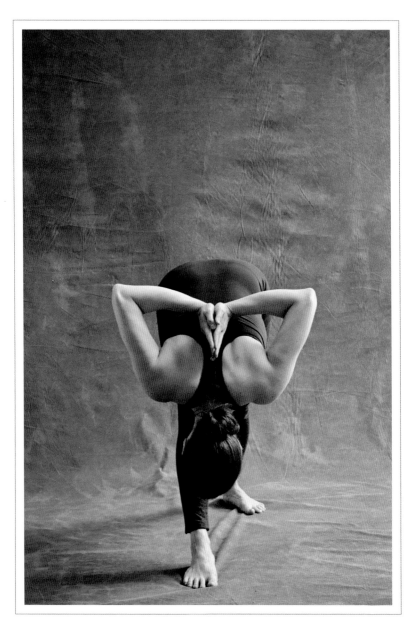

PICK YOUR PRACTICE

If you're new to yoga, here's a quick rundown of some styles likely to be available at studios or gyms near you. Vinyasa, or flow yoga, is a fluid practice that connects one movement to another in a graceful progression; choreography and challenge levels vary from class to class. Ashtanga is a very rigorous style that also connects postures in a flow, but there's no variation to the class—every single Ashtanga class consists of the same poses in the same order. In Iyengar yoga, each pose is separate (no flow), and you're likely to stay in poses for a long time; Iyengar has a very strong emphasis on alignment, so it's a great choice if you have injuries or other limitations. It's nice to sample more than one style, if multiples are available, so you can find the one that really speaks to you.

STOP IF IT HURTS

Is there a body part that chronically aches? Does one element of your exercise drill fill you with dread? Is there a gentler form of movement you're drawn to? Many of us have an almost religious commitment to our routines, despite the fact that they might be harming us. Taking things down a notch or cutting out parts that are damaging makes exercise more sustainable and enjoyable and therefore more effective. A simple rule: If something hurts, *stop doing it*.

BABY YOUR INJURIES

Maybe you have some physical therapy exercises you're supposed to be doing but aren't. We tend to treat tasks like these as homework. But if you can change your mind and think of them as indulgences—something nice you can do to care for your body, like taking a hot bath—you might be more inclined to keep up with them. It's one of those cases where we have the power to heal ourselves, if only we'll make ourselves the priority. Think about being 90. You don't want to be saying, "Ack, I should have done those darned stretches. Then maybe I wouldn't have this chronic pain in my hamstring."

DON'T LET YOUR COMPUTER WRECK YOUR SPINE

As you probably know from experience, when you're working on a computer, especially a laptop, gradually your eyes get closer to the screen, your chin juts, your back rounds, and your shoulders lift. What you might *not* know is that this posture overstretches the back muscles and shortens the connective tissue in the front of the body. Over time, your body memorizes this unhealthy collapsed misalignment as its new way of being. (It gets stuck that way!) Fixing this posture uncrushes your lungs, muscles, and organs and ups your energy level (because you'll be able to breathe better). Elevate your computer so the screen is at eye level or just above and make sure your elbows and hands are on one plane. Use a pillow under a laptop if it's in your actual lap or set it on a stand that angles the keyboard down toward your hands.

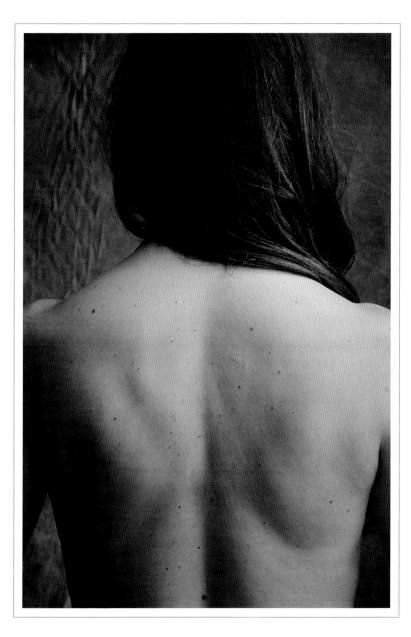

TIPTOE (DON'T BOLT) OUT OF INERTIA

If you don't yet exercise at all, be gentle as you begin. Don't start in the gym. Start in real life: Take the long way to the train in the morning, the stairs instead of the elevator. Ease yourself into movement. Then introduce more physically challenging activity. You need to wake up your body before you start lifting weights or running. When you take the drama out of it ("I'm joining the gym!"), it's easier to start. Put down this book and go for a walk.

MOVE FIVE MINUTES OUT OF EVERY HOUR

This is easy to say and hard for some to do, but make it a goal—in fact, write it on a Post-it and stick it anywhere you get stuck (at your computer, say). After 55 minutes of work, get up and walk around or climb a flight of stairs. Or if you have a private office, run through a couple of yoga poses or some old-school calisthenics (push-ups, jumping jacks)—anything that shakes you out of the "chair" shape your body's been holding. This break also gives your mind a restart, so this habit can be great for productivity.

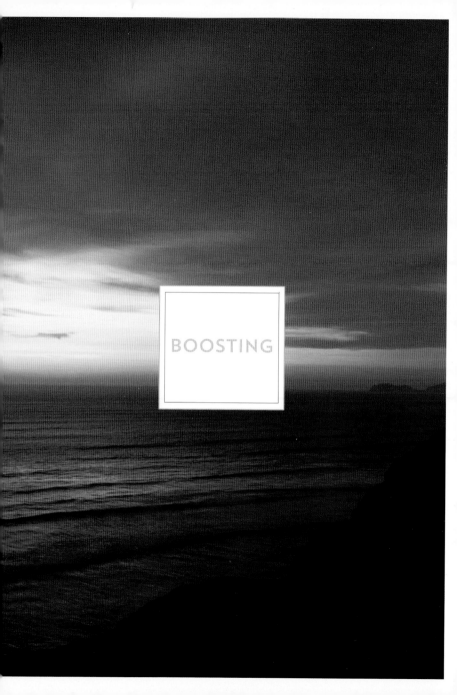

BOOSTING

GET 15 MINUTES OF SUNSHINE A DAY

Your body needs vitamin D, which comes from the sun, to protect it from all sorts of diseases, including many types of cancer. Most of us get only about half the vitamin D we need. Get out in the sun, arms and legs exposed (weather permitting) for 15 minutes every day, no sunscreen. It'll do wonders for your mood and energy level, too.

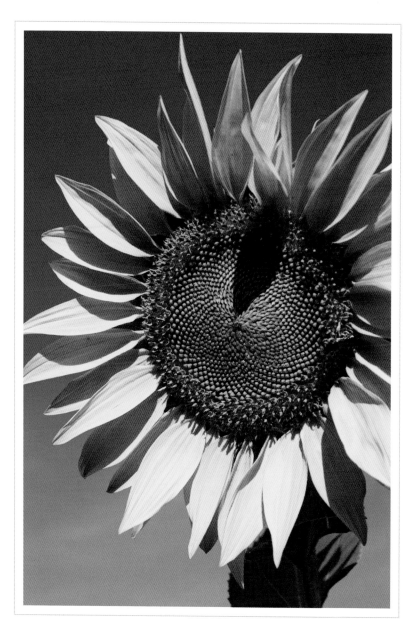

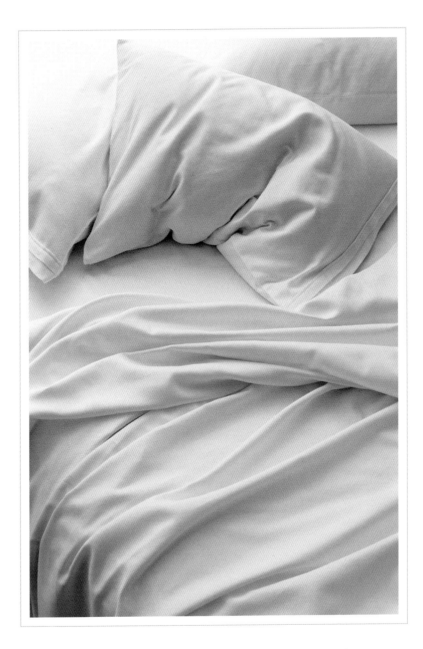

SIMPLE SECRETS FOR A GOOD NIGHT'S SLEEP

You need four things: a cool room (60° to 68°F); no screens an hour prior to bedtime (that means no TV, laptop, e-reader, phone); total darkness (don't even turn on the light in the middle of the night to go to the bathroom—it messes with your body's production of the sleep hormone melatonin); and no food or drink two hours before bedtime. That's all. Tuck in your devices in another room to keep the eerie charging lights away from your sleep zone. If you can't, use an eye mask.

SPEND LOTS OF TIME WITH PEOPLE YOU LOVE

It's a health factor, yes—a boost for your immune system. You need to be around those who really get you, to laugh, talk unguardedly about your problems, and listen deeply. You need hugs and smiles and belly laughs. You need to be able to be your true self. If you're lucky, this stuff is built into your day. But even if it requires an effort, make it happen. Don't assume e-mail or Facebook or even the phone is going to do—physical, as well as emotional, closeness is a big deal.

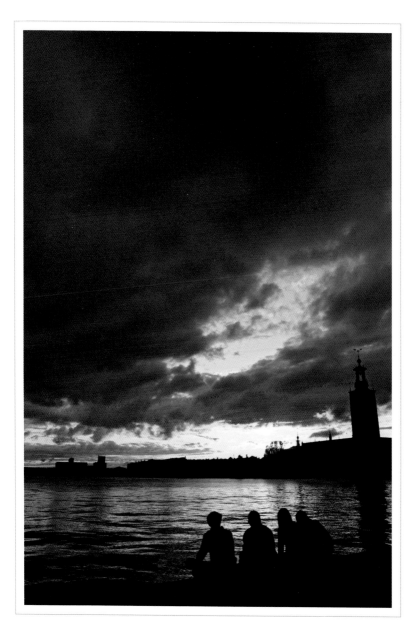

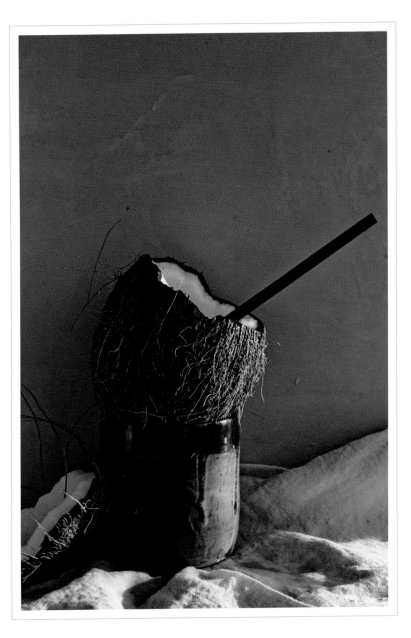

DON'T BELIEVE THE POWER-DRINK HYPE

Get your kids (and yourself) off the blue-green-orange glowing stuff. Coconut water replaces electrolytes too and is chemical free (though it has a fair amount of naturally occurring sugar, so don't overdo it). You can also swap in coconut water for plain water in a protein shake, for more flavor.

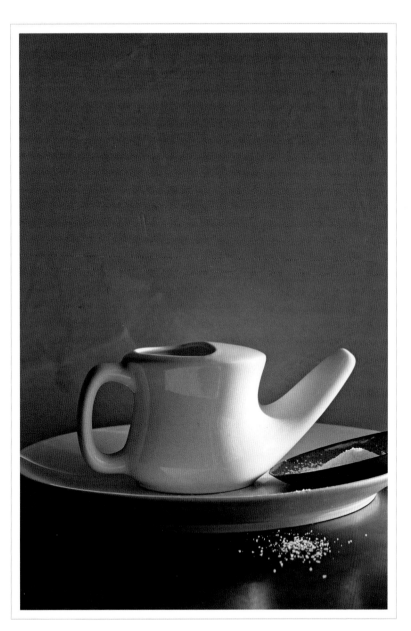

EMBRACE THE NETI POT

It's not necessarily something you want to do in front of your significant other, but neti-ing, like flossing, is a two-minute-a-day habit that quickly becomes second nature. Once you start, you'll wonder how you lived without it. If the practice seems weird or mysterious, here's all it is: You put a tiny spoonful of non-iodized salt in the pot (the spoon is included with the neti salts, or you can get premeasured packets), fill the pot with warm water, and pour the water into one nostril. Tilting your head just so, you're able to direct the water out the opposite nostril as you pour. Blow your nose, then do the other side. You'll breathe more easily, find that colds don't last as long, and lighten the impact of seasonal allergies. Watch a video online for technique. You'll have it down in no time.

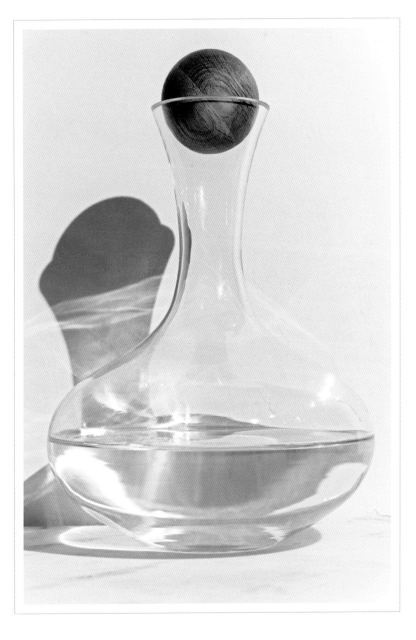

SORRY, RED WINE IS NOT MEDICINAL

You've probably heard that one glass of red wine a day is good for your body. The reason is it gives you a bit of resveratrol, a powerful antioxidant and anti-inflammatory. Don't shoot the messenger, but the truth is that the amount of resveratrol supplied by a glass of wine (1 milligram) is not significant (if a glass contained 5 milligrams, that would be a different story). Alcohol is liquid sugar. It's more depleting than restorative. To feel your best, you shouldn't be having alcohol every day, even red wine.

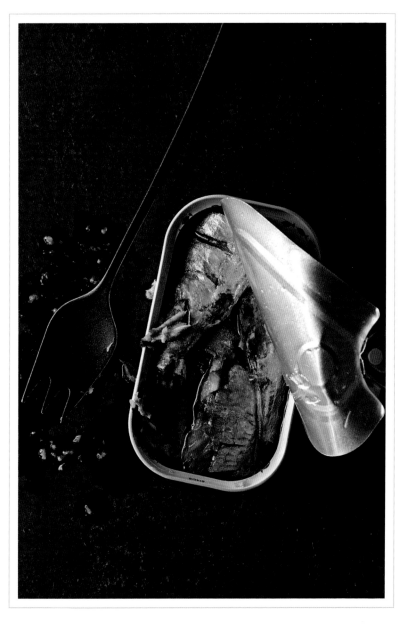

WHAT ARE OMEGA-3S, AND WHY DO THEY MATTER?

Omega-3s are healthy fats your body needs: They lower your cholesterol and your blood pressure; strengthen your immune system; boost the health of your brain, joints, heart, and eyes; and reduce inflammation (which is connected with all sorts of diseases). Great sources are wild salmon, walnuts, grass-fed meat, ground flaxseeds, and sardines.

WHY BOTHER WITH SUPPLEMENTS?

In a perfect world, our soil would have plenty of vital nutrients, and the produce at your grocery store would be packed with all the minerals and vitamins you need. But that's just not our reality anymore— our soil is depleted, and even when we eat lots of fresh, organic food, we're still lacking certain nutrients. Supplements, as the name indicates, add what's missing. They fill in the gaps, even for those who are making the best possible food choices.

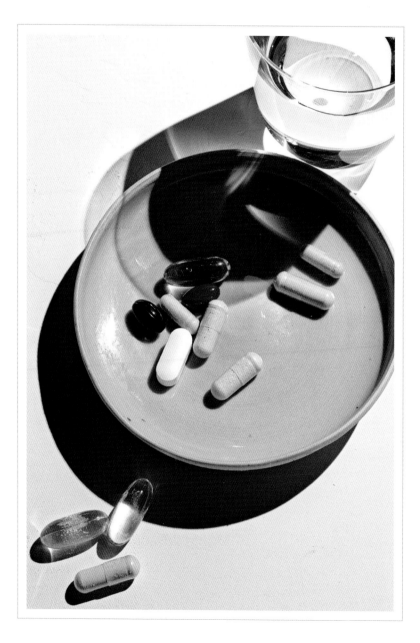

TAKE THESE EVERY DAY

MULTIVITAMIN

Choose a multi meant to be taken twice a day (one-a-day types generally can't fit in enough of what you need). Buy them in capsule, not tablet, form—they're easier for your body to break down. Get a natural version, without sugar, lactose, or artificial colors. If you see magnesium oxide (a cheap and less nutritious form of magnesium) on the label, it's probably not a good-quality vitamin. Quality is a big issue when it comes to all supplements.

VITAMIN D

Even if you get plenty of sunshine, there's a good chance you could use more vitamin D (see page 136)—especially in the winter, when the sun is low and we spend less time outside. Deficiencies are associated with cancer, heart disease, high blood pressure, arthritis, Parkinson's, and Alzheimer's. Make sure your supplement contains D3 (not D2), and check with your doctor on the right dosage for your levels.

OMEGA-3 FISH OIL

High-quality fish oil is kind of a magic potion, lowering your risk of heart disease and lessening inflammation, which protects you from type 2 diabetes and arthritis. It also helps with depression, anxiety, and exhaustion. Check to make sure the fish oil you buy has been tested for mercury.

PROBIOTICS

Doctors have finally caught on that antibiotics are depleting our bodies of essential bacteria and now recommend taking a probiotic to balance the gut when they prescribe antibiotics. But to maintain the level of good bacteria we really need, we should be taking probiotics every day, not just when we're on antibiotics. The probiotics you should buy are usually kept in the fridge (not on the shelf) and should contain at least 20 billion viable bacteria per serving. Some people think if they eat a lot of yogurt, they're getting the probiotics they need. But commercial yogurts are not a good source of probiotics; pasteurization kills most of the good bacteria.

TAKE THESE IF YOU NEED THEM

If you have very low blood pressure, take licorice root extract—150 milligrams twice a day. It's a natural boost for the adrenal glands, which are related to low blood pressure. (Don't take it if you have normal or high blood pressure.)

If you're a vegan or a strict vegetarian, take B12, which comes from organ meat, fish, eggs, and dairy and helps keep your energy up. Also take B12 if you're over 65 (even if you're a meat-eater), because the body's ability to absorb the vitamins in food starts to decline as we age.

If you're not sleeping well, take magnesium glycinate at bedtime. It also helps regulate blood pressure, strengthen joints, keep the immune system strong, and support your heart and your brain.

STEP AWAY FROM THE STATINS

If you're on a statin drug like Lipitor to lower your cholesterol, you may know there's controversy surrounding these meds. Here's clarity: Lowering cholesterol does *not*, it turns out, prevent heart attacks and strokes. We've been sold a bill of goods. The big deal about this is that millions of people are on statins unnecessarily, and statins cause diabetes, liver damage, nervous system problems, muscle weakness, and more. Talk to your doctor about possibly getting off statins. And in the meantime, if you're taking statins, also take 200 mg of co-enzyme Q10 daily; it helps minimize side effects like weakness and muscle pain.

THE POWER OF CHIA

These tiny seeds with a mild taste (a little like that of poppy seeds) deliver a whopping dose of nutrients, especially omega-3s. They also make you feel fuller faster, which is a plus if you're trying to lose weight. Sprinkle on nut butter or add to a shake. Or make a delicious, creamy pudding: Mix one can of full-cream coconut milk (Native Forest is a great brand) with 2 tablespoons of chia seeds, 2 tablespoons of raw cacao, and a pinch of stevia to sweeten. Stir it up well, then place it in the fridge, and in 10 minutes you'll have a rich, chocolatey dessert.

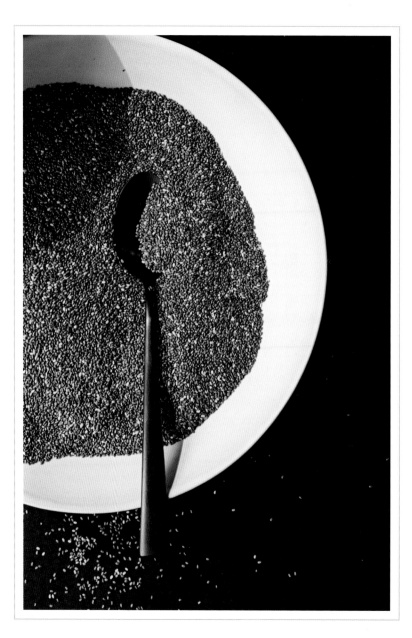

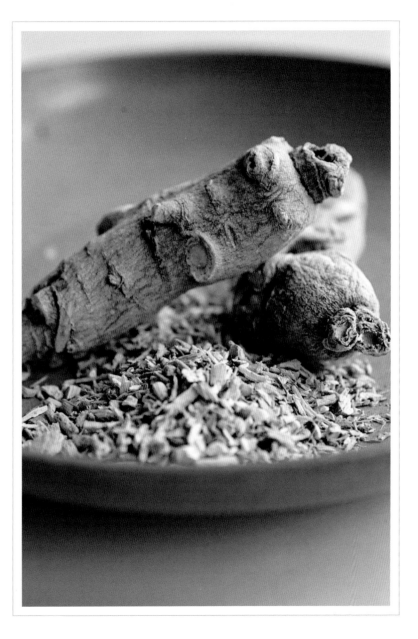

FORTIFY YOUR ADRENALS

The crazy lives most of us live—perpetually multi-tasking, staying "on" even when we're not at work, doing too much too often, and grabbing carbs and caffeine because we're too busy for a proper meal—do a real number on the adrenal glands. These glands are meant to control how we react to stress, but when we live in a constant state of low-grade stress, as so many of us do, they get exhausted. Then they signal the thyroid for help and it too becomes depleted, which messes with our metabolism and makes us gain weight. If you're feeling generally and inexplicably crummy, it could be that your adrenal glands and thyroid have just about had it with your current patterns. There are herbal supplements that help, called adaptogens. Take them daily for three months, then give your body a month off. Make sure the formulas you choose contain Asian ginseng, eleuthero, ashwagandha, and *Rhodiola rosea*.

LEARN YOUR NUMBERS

Next time you make an appointment with your doctor, ask to have the following checked: your vitamin D, your hemoglobin A1C, and your fasting blood glucose. Many doctors don't take these numbers seriously enough. Vitamin D should be at least 40. If it's not, you need supplements. Hemoglobin A1C should be 5.5 or lower, and fasting blood glucose should be below 95. If either is off, your body may not be processing sugar properly (this includes fruit, bread, pasta, even sugary vegetables like beets). In this case, switch to a low-carb Paleo diet.

RETHINK YOUR DOCTORS

If you like the advice in this book, you might want to look for a functional medicine practitioner for yourself and your family. Functional medicine doctors focus on finding root causes, not just medicating symptoms. They look at the whole patient and see each patient as an individual. Basically, having a functional medicine doctor gives you a partner in your health journey. You can trust that someone is looking at the big picture for you. To find a well-trained practitioner near you, go to functionalmedicine.org.

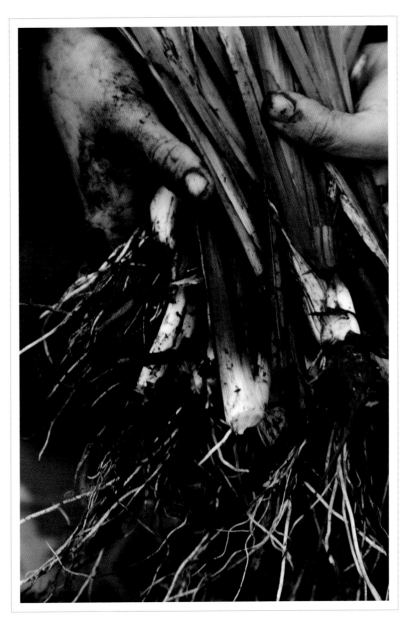

GET YOUR HANDS DIRTY

Your body needs microbes from outdoors to keep your immune system strong. Most of us live way too much of our lives inside (house, car, office), often inhaling processed air. So dig in the garden, play in the sand, and do cartwheels on the lawn whenever you can.

RESPECT YOUR INTERNAL CLOCK

Not that life will always cooperate, but when you understand your patterns of appetite and energy, you can kind of hack in there and help yourself. If you know, for instance, that there's a sweets craving coming at 4:00 P.M. that drives you, zombielike, to the office vending machine, get some fresh air at 3:00, and see if that heads off the craving. Likewise if the stress of work gives you energy to burn, exercising in the evening might make more sense than working out in the morning. While we're all individual, we share certain patterns. Many of us have a period of intellectual clarity early in the day, after sleep gently cleanses our brains. (Ever wake up with a "eureka" moment?) Maybe you can adjust your schedule to take advantage of "morning mind"— tackling an intellectual or creative challenge before the concerns of the day fill up your head.

ENERGY BARS
SAP YOUR STRENGTH

They don't belong in your kids' lunches—they're full of sugar—and you shouldn't be eating them regularly either. As a rare treat or in an emergency, have a bar from one of the less-processed brands like Kind or Lara. When you're grabbing something at a deli, make it raw nuts instead. And get in the habit of keeping some protein shake packets in your bag or desk drawer so you can get a *real* energy boost when you need it.

DON'T BE AFRAID OF ACUPUNCTURE

For muscle pain, digestive trouble, insomnia, headaches, and more, acupuncture can be really effective. The basic thinking is that the body has a system of meridians—imagine tiny rivers—through which vital energy flows. When something goes wrong, it's an indication that there's a block in the system. Acupuncture restores flow. Acupuncture needles are much finer than needles used to deliver medicine—they're flexible, not rigid. And they're sterile and disposable. Often you don't feel them at all. But depending on the spot and the tension in that spot, it may hurt for a few seconds when a needle goes in. Once the needles are placed, you relax for a while—could be 15 minutes, could be 45; sometimes there's calming music playing—then the practitioner removes the needles, which you won't even feel. Find a good practitioner through a friend or a doctor you trust, and if you're nervous, book a consultation first.

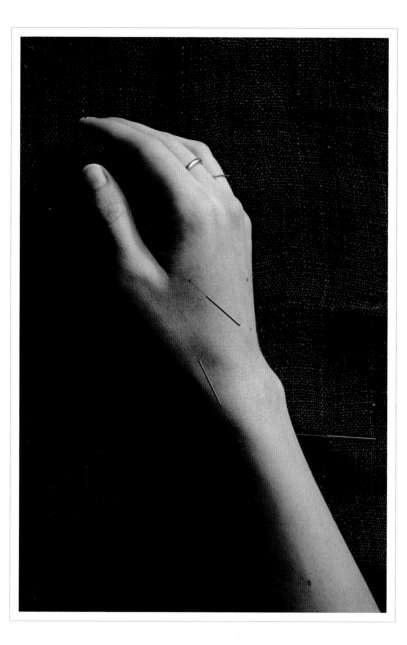

LOOK UP

Be present in your surroundings. Looking up and out—and making eye contact with others—is a form of nourishment that the age of smartphones has seriously messed with. See the sky, look at the ticket collector on the commuter train, take note of the people nearby when you're eating lunch. Instead of burying your face in your phone—which takes you out of the moment and often into a sort of junk-food-for-the-eye place—lift your head and be part of your environment.

RESET YOUR BACK

After a long day at the office, or whenever you feel achy and crooked, you can use a foam roller (the kind you might have seen at the gym or Pilates studio) to give yourself an adjustment. Sit on the floor and place the roller behind you, with one end at your tailbone. Lower yourself back, lying down with your spine along the roller. Keep your knees bent and feet flat for now so you can easily adjust yourself. Let your arms drape comfortably to the side and relax your weight into the roller. Breathe and stay there for about five minutes. Then roll to one side, remove the roller, and lie flat on the floor for another minute or two.

JUST SAY NO (THANKS)

Many of us are packed to the gills with obligations and activities, largely out of habit. We say yes to things we could probably politely refuse and end up exhausted. As an experiment, try cutting your load of optional commitments in half. See what happens when your schedule isn't jam-packed. With a little air in it, your concentration, productivity, and efficiency are likely to improve. You'll also probably feel happier and more satisfied.

SLEEP-TRAIN YOURSELF

It's hard to imagine going to bed and getting up at the same time every day, with weekdays so demanding and weekends used for refueling. But if you reinforce a rhythm—say 11:30 bedtime and 6:30 wake-up—your body will help you out. It will learn to start producing melatonin at around 11:00, to make you sleepy. And at around 6:00, it'll start pumping wake-up hormones, serotonin and cortisol. Falling asleep and waking up will both be less of an effort. (Even when you aren't able to get to bed at the usual hour, do your best to stick with your wake-up time.)

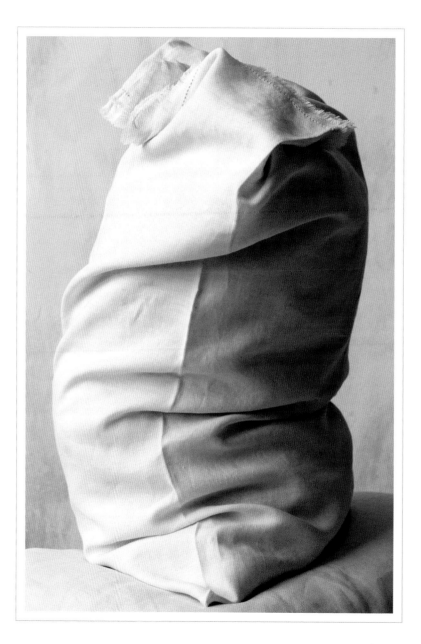

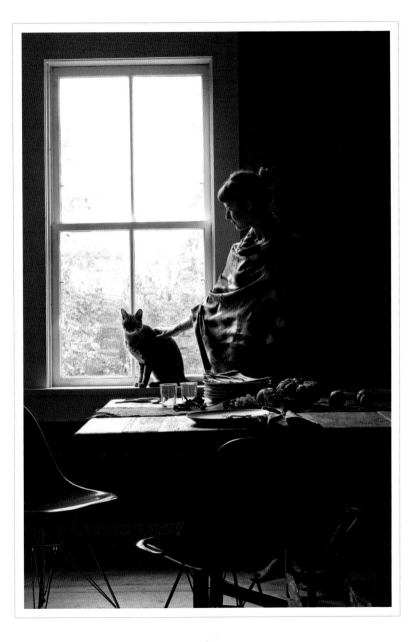

ADOPT A KITTEN

Or a puppy. Or a nice old animal that doesn't ask for more than a little love. People with pets live longer, on average, than those without. And stroking a cat or petting a dog releases serotonin, your brain's happy chemical. Feng shui likes pets because they move energy—they keep a space alive. Find a shelter near you at aspca.org.

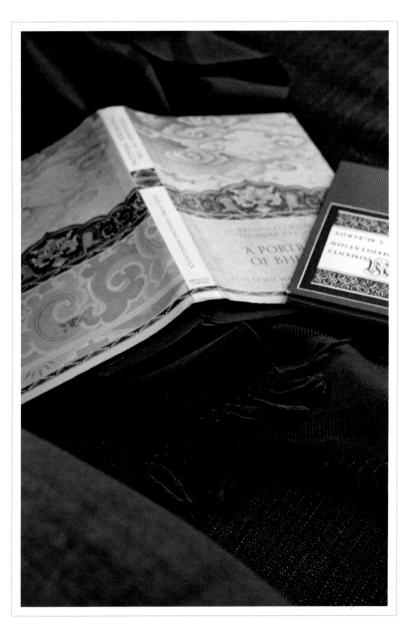

SOLO-TASK

We've all heard that multitasking is ineffective, and yet the speed of our lives has us piling one thing on top of another as a matter of course. One nice way to quiet the chatter in your head is to give your whole focus to an everyday task. While doing the laundry, just do the laundry: Listen to the sound of the water as it fills the washing machine, notice the smell of the detergent, feel the clothes in your hand. Make it a very casual moving meditation. It doesn't take up any more time than it would when done with your mind darting every which way or your phone pressed to your ear—you don't have to move in slow motion. But intentional awareness slows the mind, brings a feeling of calm, and allows insights to bubble up (one of which might be that it's really satisfying and enjoyable to focus on one thing at a time). Take that to work and you'll see a difference.

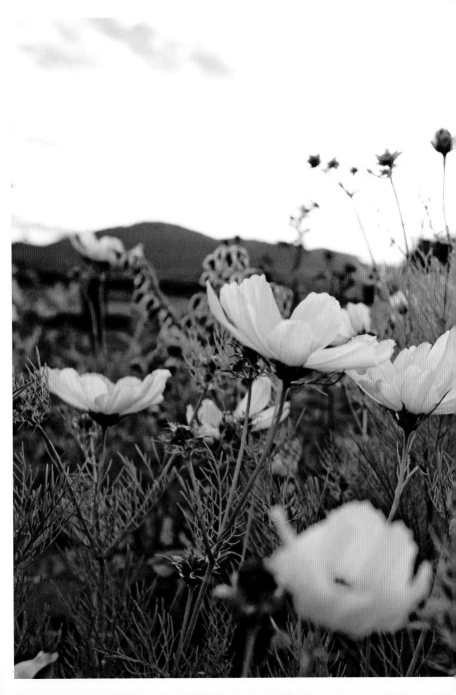

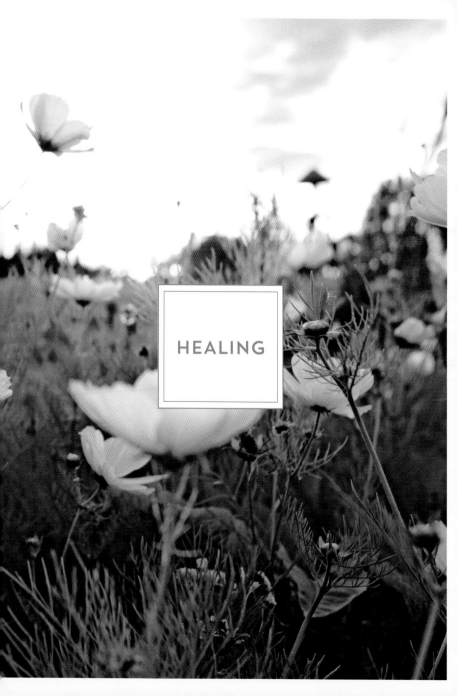

HEALING

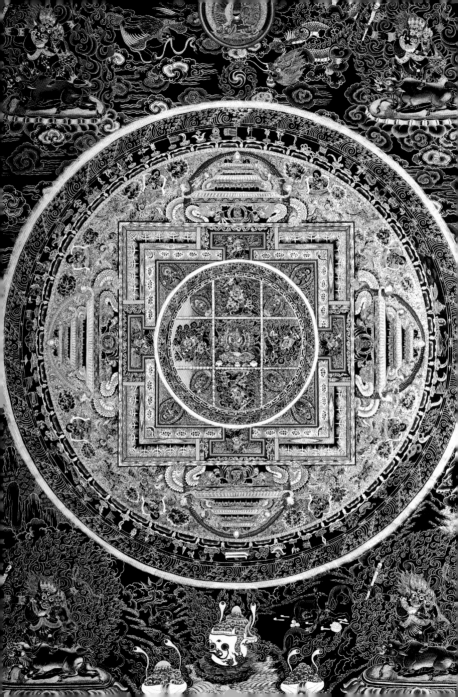

WHY MEDITATION IS WORTH IT

Meditation triggers a relaxation cycle in the body—oxygen in, tension out—that not only feels great but also changes the way you react to stress. When you meditate regularly, you'll find that small irritations and big challenges don't hit you as hard as they used to; you're a little calmer, and a little nicer. On a practical level, meditation gives you a great place to put your overactive mind when you're replaying events or feeling anxious about what's to come. Think of it as a wholesome alternative to a stiff drink. There are different types of practices—some loose and others structured. Take any opportunity to try them and find what works for you. Once you get into it, meditation is like a tool you have in your back pocket. You can use it anytime, anywhere, to rest, relax, and restart.

SWITCH THE LENS

Many of us are conditioned to worry and complain. Fretting sometimes feels like a tax we have to pay to remain relatively safe and sound—and our bodies play along, converting stress into pain. "Think positive" may sound hollow, but the health benefits of looking on the bright side are massive. If you're reading this book, you probably have all the basics— shelter, food, water, a community of people who care about you. So next time you find yourself indulging in the habit of negative thinking ("I hate this traffic," "I'll never get out of this job," "Why can't I meet someone already?"), reframe your thinking—find a silver lining or focus on something you're grateful for. When you switch the lens and heal your mind of negativity, it actually helps heal your body of exhaustion, aches, and pains.

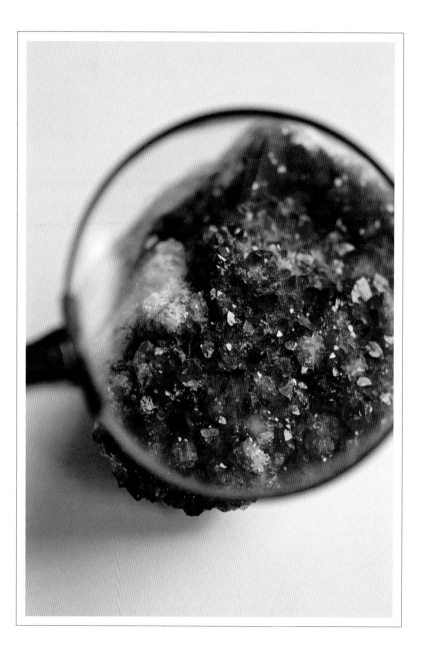

DO SOMETHING YOU LOVE FOR AT LEAST 10 MINUTES A DAY

It's incredibly powerful and healing. We all think we don't have time, but most of us can find it somewhere (maybe in the time we spend online—just a guess). It doesn't have to be a big deal: Shoot hoops in the driveway. Sketch something on the bus home. Blast music and dance around the living room. Pick up an instrument and play three pieces. Do it on purpose, like taking a supplement.

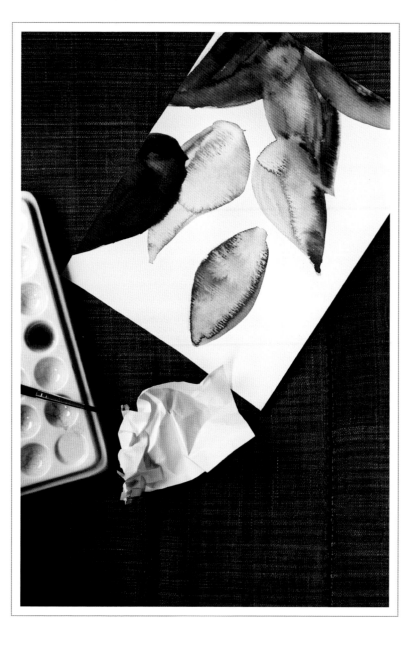

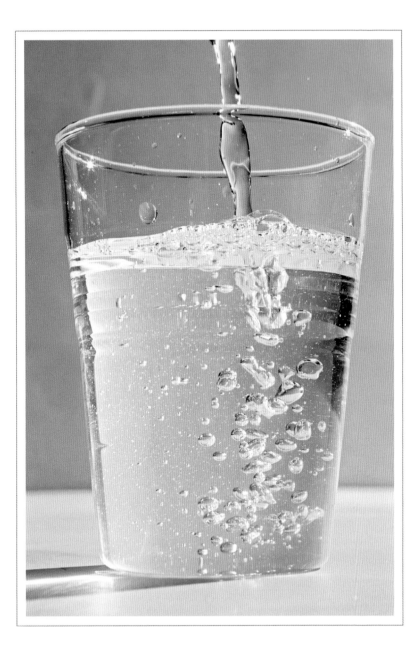

MAKE WATER YOUR DEFAULT BEVERAGE

You probably don't have to count glasses as long as water is generally what you reach for. Your thirst mechanism will tell you when you need it. And we all need it, to keep the digestive system and kidneys functioning smoothly and to hydrate skin (among other things). But if you're not in the habit of drinking water, follow the old rule of about eight glasses a day. To lessen your caffeine load, occasionally replace your morning drink with water (cold or hot) plus a generous squeeze of lemon (don't drop citrus into the glass, though, unless it's organic and washed).

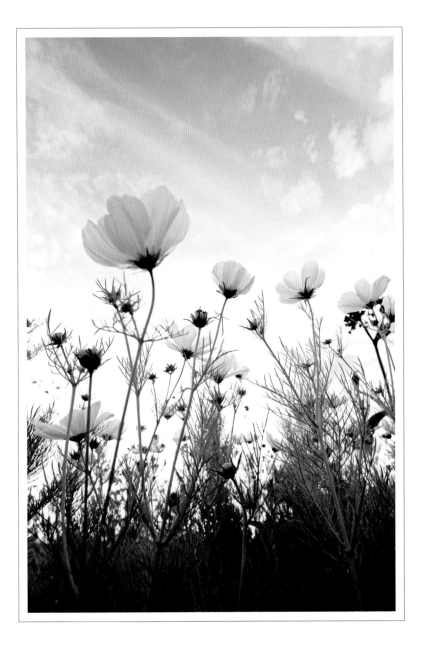

WANDER BAREFOOT

Kick off your shoes and walk on grass, earth, or sand whenever you have the chance. Not only will this boost your immune system by exposing you to unfamiliar microbes, but it will also give you a little charge—literally. Believe it or not, just as we get vitamin D from the sun and oxygen from the air, we get electrons from the earth, which have calming and healing benefits for the whole body.

TAKE A VACATION FROM SCREENS

Those who remember life before addictive electronic devices need no explanation of why it's important to break away from technology regularly. For the younger set: Think of it as a cleanse for your mind. After some discomfort and craving, you'll discover a clarity and peace you may never have known.

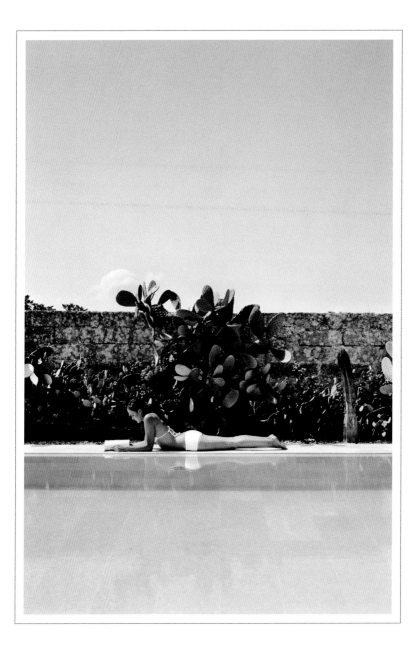

HONOR THY FEET

They're the command center of the body. Be nice to them. While you're doing dishes or chitchatting on the phone, roll a tennis ball under the bottom of one foot, then the other, for five minutes each (or to really spoil yourself, use a foot roller). It ungrips all the tiny muscles that hold up your frame all day and has gentle trickle-up benefits for your entire system. Minimize the number of hours you spend in torturous shoes. High heels don't just hurt your feet; they affect the body all the way up—knees, hips, spine, neck (and then your brain and mood, because if you're hurting, you're cranky). When you take off a pair, always take two minutes (literally *two minutes*) to stretch yourself back into shape; stand on a step with just the balls of your feet and let one heel lower down for a deep calf stretch. Hold for a few seconds, then switch feet. Repeat 10 times.

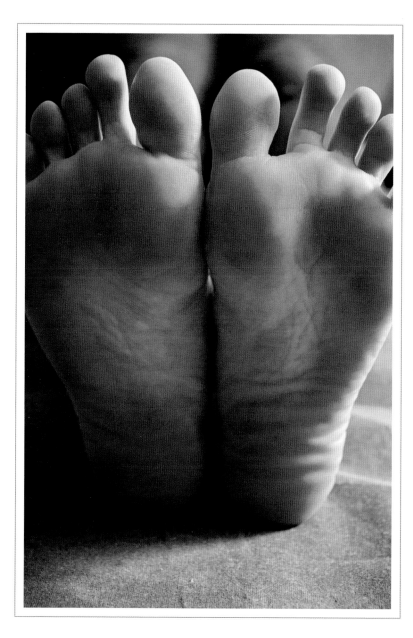

TAKE FOOD SENSITIVITIES SERIOUSLY

Maybe you have a vague sense that you don't process dairy well or that gluten is a problem, but you've never really isolated it to find out—either because it seems like a pain in the neck or because you don't really want to know. But it's better to know and to feel good all the time than to suffer stomachaches and weariness: For two weeks, cut out gluten (pasta, bread), dairy, corn, soy, sugar, and anything else you suspect you might be sensitive to. Then reintroduce foods one at a time, with two days in between. On test day, have a heaping helping of the food in question for breakfast and then again at lunch—you'll get a really clear read on how your body reacts to it.

CONSIDER A DIETARY DETOX

Your body has its own cleaning system that's working all the time to fight toxins you take in through air, water, and processed foods; it's also battling toxins that come from the inside (an unbalanced gut can produce a lot of toxins). When this system gets overloaded, you feel bloated, congested, achy, and exhausted. A dietary detox (or a cleanse—same thing) helps by boosting your body's own detox system and fortifying your gut and liver. Take a detox supplement that includes antimicrobial and antiparasitic herbs like black walnut hull, bernerine, grapefruit seed extract, wormwood, and bearberry. For the liver, look for supplements with quercetin, milk thistle, and dandelion. For two weeks, drop sugar, wheat, alcohol, dairy, caffeine, soy, corn, fried foods, and packaged foods from your diet, and take your detox supplements. You'll feel amazing. Twice a year is great, but more often is fine too.

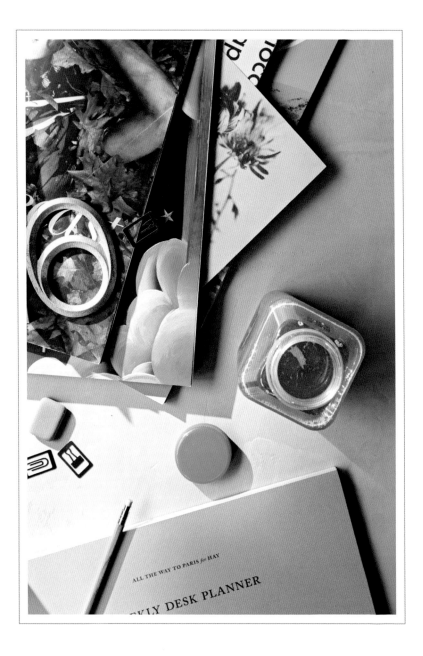

A JUICE FAST
IS NOT A DETOX

The point of a juice fast is not to nourish your body, it's to rest your digestive system. There's nothing wrong with it, as long as you're juicing mostly green vegetables (not fruits—too much sugar!). But you'll probably feel very hungry consuming nothing but liquid, and that can make you really crabby. Also keep in mind that any weight you lose while juice-fasting will likely reappear as soon as you start eating again.

MUSIC CAN WORK LIKE MEDITATION

Think of the way you feel when you're sitting on a beach. Your body's rhythms—including the duration of a breath and the speed of your heartbeat—conform to the pulse of the waves. In everyday life, the noise around us (traffic and construction and leaf blowers and barking dogs) affects the vibrating atoms in our cells. Soothing music slows down our internal rhythms and stimulates the parasympathetic system, our built-in calmer (just like meditation). If you're just learning to meditate and you're struggling with the silence, relaxing with your favorite mellow music is a more accessible option.

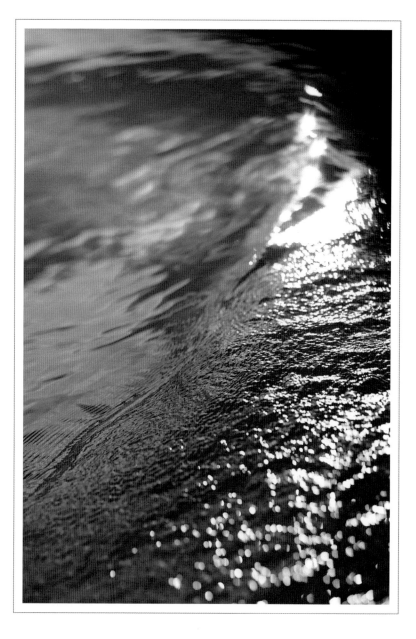

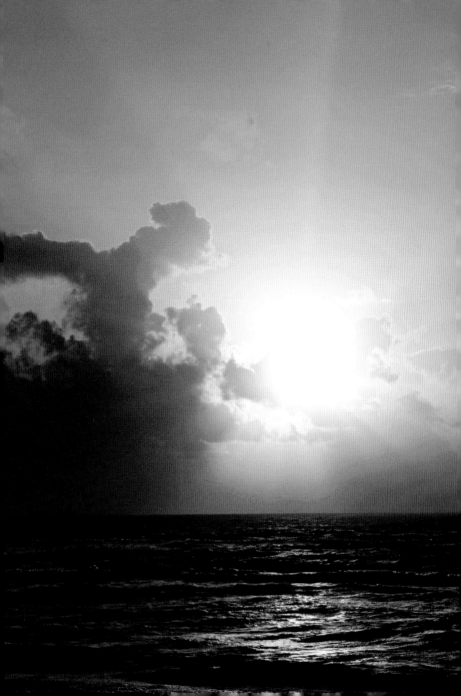

LINK WITH THE SUN

Most of us get too much light at night, when we need darkness to trigger melatonin production, and too little natural light during the day, because we're trapped inside under fluorescents. Try rising with the sun and stepping outside first thing, even just for a minute or two, to let your body feel the day-light. Find a time in the day (the earlier, the better) when you can be exposed to natural light for at least a half hour. At night, dim the lights at home; when you go to bed, remember to make the room totally dark (cover digital clock lights in your room). Chances are, you'll fall asleep more easily and sleep more soundly.

LIGHTEN YOUR LOAD

We're all seventh graders when it comes to the bag we carry. We want to look cool. But sporting a heavy bag on one shoulder all the time makes you crooked and causes a slow build of injury. You might notice it in the opposite knee, hip, low back, and shoulder (as in, if you carry your bag on the right, the left side hurts). Ultimately, of course, it's a lot sexier to be able to walk upright, loosely and gracefully, than to be hunched and in chronic pain due to years of lugging your (silly-heavy) bag.

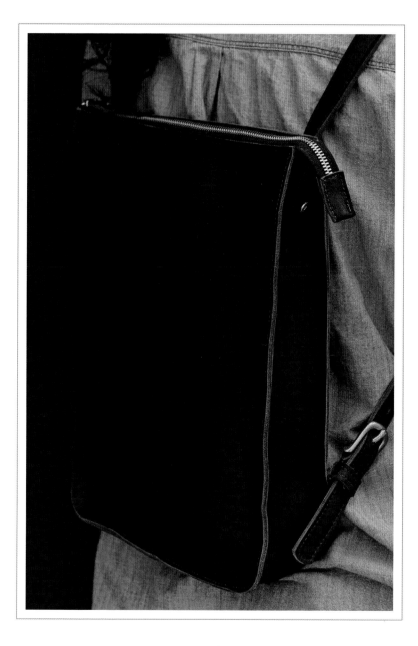

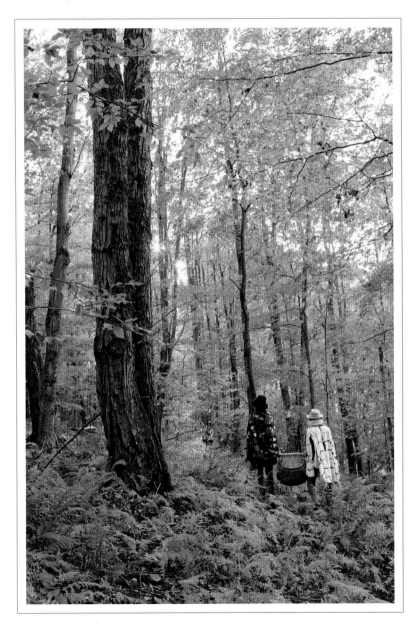

BE UNPRODUCTIVE

Sometimes the organ that needs the most care and restoration is the brain. If you're a very driven person who has no patience for an unproductive day, what you might really need is . . . an unproductive day. No to-do list. No phone. No computer. It's akin to giving your muscles a day off from weight training to rebuild and come back stronger. If a whole day seems nuts, make it a couple of hours and do something that seems like a complete waste of time. Take an easy walk on flat ground, sit on the lawn with a book, or people-watch in a café.

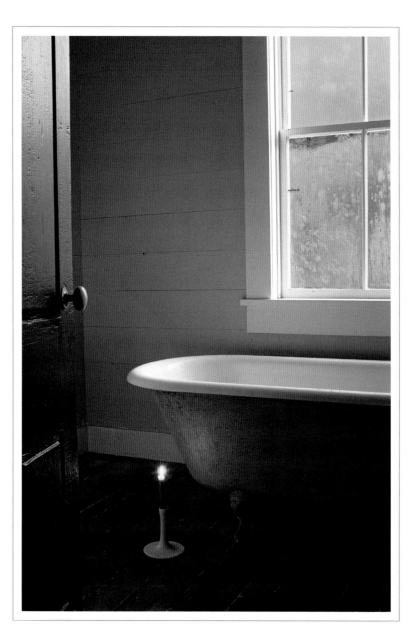

GET READY FOR BED AN HOUR EARLIER

Maybe this means sacrificing a ritual you love—plopping down on the couch with a juicy TV show after the dishes are done and/or the kids are in bed. But give it a go. Take a bath, do a relaxing yoga pose, or, if you're not tired at all, sit in a comfy chair with a book. If you're totally beat, climb into bed with said book. One of the reasons we all accept feeling crummy is that we know we don't get enough sleep. So see what happens when you do. Your mind is likely to be clearer and sharper, your mood will be better, and you'll have more patience and energy and joy.

DO SOMETHING BESIDES WORK AND PLAY

Helping others, working for a cause you connect with, participating in something that sparks your compassion and passion, is not just an important part of being human; it's an important part of being *healthy*. When you engage in something that matters to you, your spirit and energy surge (sort of the way they do when you're in love). You feel—physically— way better. Are you shaking your head, thinking "I don't have the time"? Look at it this way: When you add something you care about, you change the way the pie chart of your life is divided. That new thing that matters finds a place in your world, and when it's let in, the things that stress you out get smaller. Investigate options. Ask friends. Poke around online. And sign up for something. There's a nice phrase that cuts through the barriers to this kind of small but significant step: "Commit. You'll figure it out."

CULTIVATE KINDNESS

Forget pay-it-forward or anything about karma. This is just about being nice and good with no expectation of reciprocity or personal gain. Let someone cut ahead of you in line, listen to someone who needs an ear, give a compliment you really mean. Make your default mode one of generosity. It's a nice way to live, and it's contagious.

LET IT GO

We naturally replay situations in our heads, especially when something has gone wrong, but after one or two rounds there's no learning, only a vortex of stress that can really beat us up. When you find yourself overruminating, notice it; jot down what's bugging you (get it out of your head and onto a piece of paper) and dive into a shared activity—a conversation, Legos with your kids, a meeting, or a book.

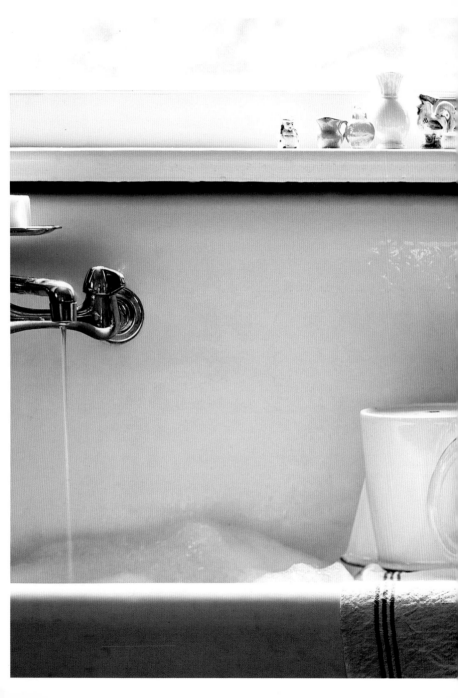

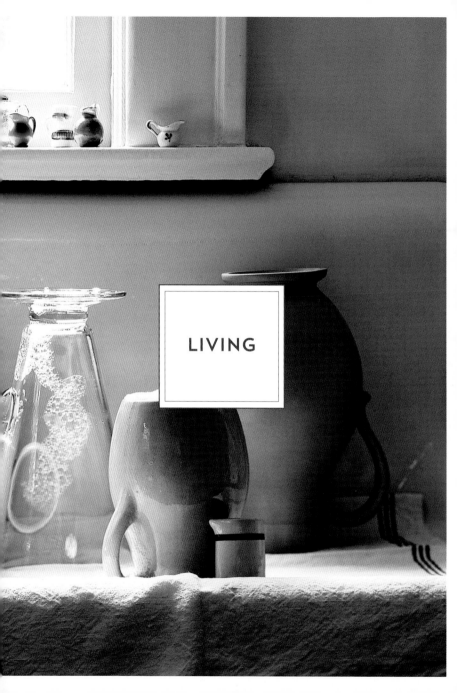

LIVING

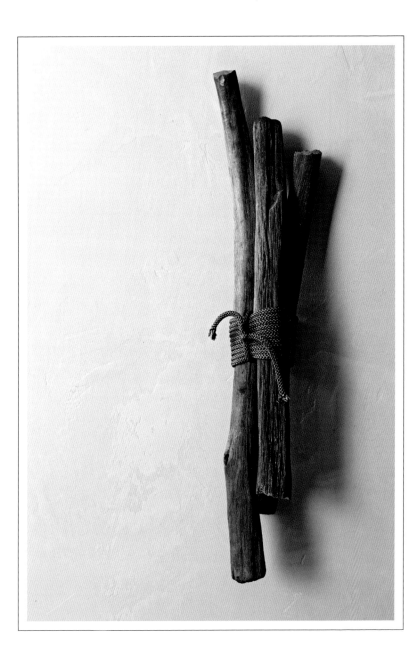

CLEAN YOUR TAP WATER

The substances added to drinking water to help "clean" it or to benefit our teeth—specifically chlorine and fluoride—are bad for the hormonal system, especially the thyroid, which controls your metabolism, among other things. Use a carbon filtration system on the kitchen sink (Aquasana's is well-priced and effective) or use natural charcoal sticks in a carafe of tap water. And install a filter for your shower.

USE HEALTHY POTS AND PANS

That means cookware made of cast iron, ceramic, or stainless steel. Copper and aluminum can leach into your food. And nonstick surfaces like Teflon contain chemicals that have been proven harmful to animals. While you're at it, get rid of plastic food-storage containers (never, ever microwave in plastic); use glass instead. And watch out for plastic water bottles, especially under the summer sun. Stainless steel or glass bottles are safer.

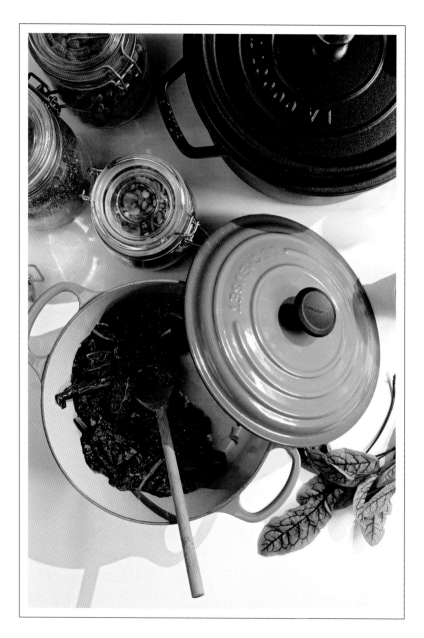

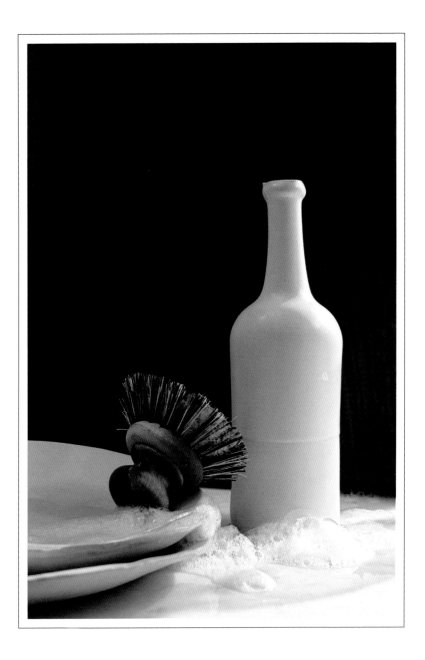

READ YOUR DISH SOAP LABEL

Some brands contain an antibacterial called triclosan. When that stuff combines with water that's been treated with chlorine (sometimes used to sanitize tap water), the result is chloroform, a potential carcinogen. Also scan the label for quaternium-15, which can release formaldehyde. Toss your dish soap if it contains either.

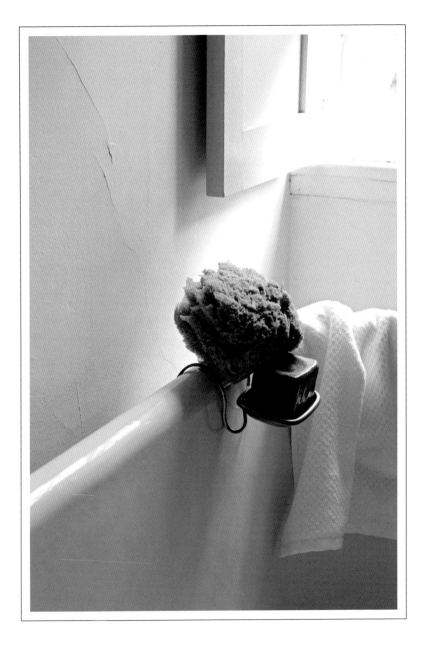

WHAT YOU PUT *ON* YOUR BODY GOES *IN* YOUR BODY

It's not just what you put in your mouth that affects your well-being. It's also the lotions, creams, soaps, hair products, and makeup you put *on* it—anything applied to your skin becomes a factor in your health. Check labels for sodium lauryl sulfate and sodium laureth sulfate. Combined with certain other chemicals, like TEA (check for that one too), they can form a carcinogen. Also scan ingredient lists for diazolidinyl urea, imidazolidinyl urea, and quaternium-15—which all release formaldehyde—and for parabens (banned in Europe because of links to cancer but still legal here). Apps like Think Dirty make it easy to assess all sorts of beauty products.

KEEP CHLORINE OUT OF THE HOUSE

Check cleaning products for bleach, sodium hypo-chlorite, hypochlorite, and chlorine. They're all essen-tially the same thing, and you don't want them in your home. Chlorine is a toxin, and it can affect your immune system, your thyroid, and your respiratory system, among other things.

DON'T USE ANTIBACTERIAL HAND SOAP

The synthetic antibacterial ingredient triclosan in many hand cleansers disrupts hormones, messes with your immune system, and can affect fertility. Break the habit of squirting antibacterial sanitizer on your hands multiple times a day, and get that antibacterial soap out of your bathroom. There's just no reason to expose yourself to the risks, when studies have shown that plain old soap and water are just as effective.

WASH THE AIR

Keep plants in the house. Open the windows when you can. Skip the AC when possible and use a fan to pull in fresh air. Dehumidify damp rooms to prevent mold. Use fresh eucalyptus instead of room spray. When you pick up your dry cleaning, forgo the plastic and hang clothes outside in the fresh air for a bit—or just walk them home uncovered—so you take fewer chemicals into your closet.

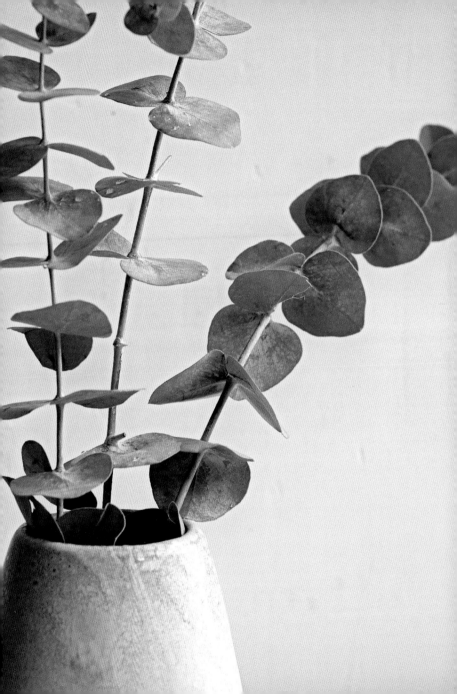

GREEN YOUR CLEANERS ONE BY ONE

Every step you take away from the toxic stuff makes your home safer. If you don't want to waste what you've already purchased, start with those that get closest to your body: dish soap (residue left on clean plates can mix with your food and end up inside you) and laundry detergent. Then, as you run out of all-purpose spray, glass cleaner, and so on, replace each with a safe, nonchemical alternative. There's a lot of vague labeling out there, so visit ewg.org for well-vetted options. Or make your own cleaners. With baking soda, white vinegar, lemons, castile soap, borax, and tea tree oil, you can concoct pretty much anything you need and never again have to worry about what might be lurking inside a commercial spray bottle.

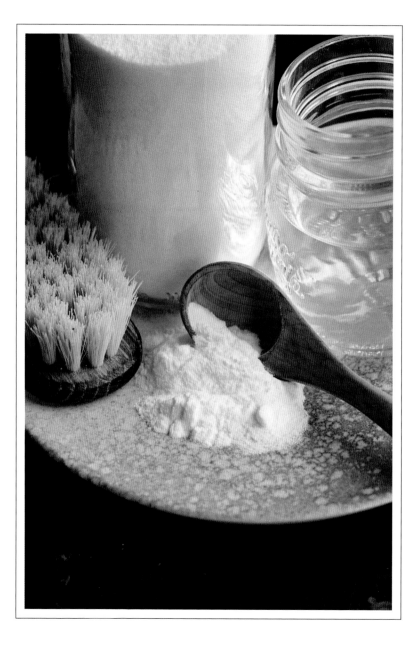

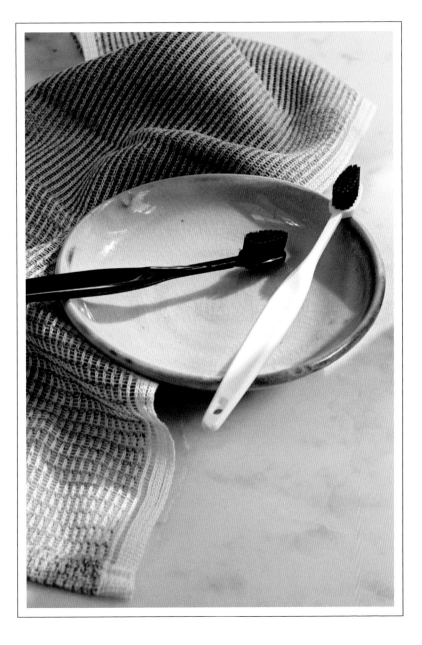

"NATURAL" TOOTHPASTE IS NOT ALWAYS NATURAL

You might think you're already using a healthful toothpaste, but hidden in some brands that slap "natural" on the packaging are dyes, artificial flavorings, and chemicals like propylene glycol, triclosan, SLS, or SLES. Check labels or switch to pure brands like Tom's of Maine or Natural Dentist. This is a critical choice, because you actually ingest bits of toothpaste. For kids it might be a tough switch, but it's an important health upgrade that could stick with them for life.

SWITCH FROM MINERAL OIL TO COCONUT OIL

Petroleum jelly, mineral oil, baby oil—they're all the same thing: a nasty petrochemical that's terrible for your body; it suffocates skin and slows its natural cell development. Use pure coconut oil or shea butter as a moisturizer or makeup remover instead. Moisturizer has a particularly hefty impact on your system: Consider the surface area it covers and the fact that the product stays on all day, permeating skin. Natural organic coconut oil is a simple solution, or go with products from beauty brands like Dr. Hauschka, Naturopathica, Soapwalla, REN, Sumbody, and CV Skinlabs, which use nothing but pure ingredients.

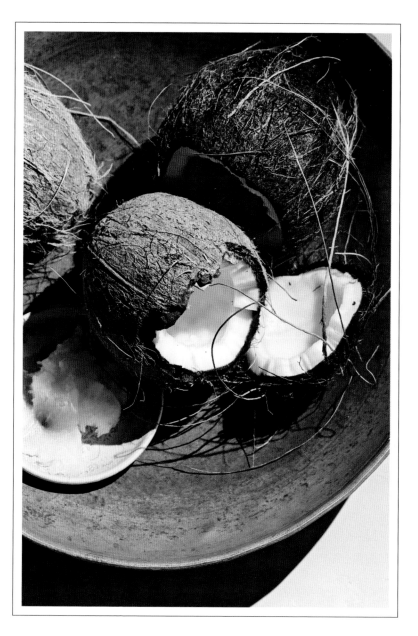

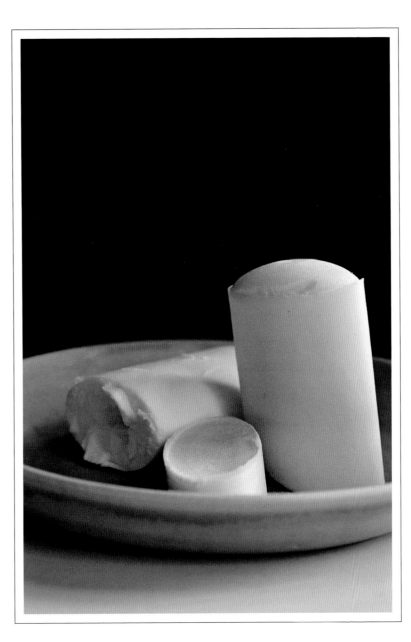

LOSE THE MAINSTREAM DEODORANT

We're all afraid of natural deodorant because we're worried it doesn't work as well. And it doesn't. You need to try a couple of brands to find the one that's most effective for you (give it time—your body needs to adjust to a chemical-free formula) and maybe get in the habit of reapplying at a certain point in the day. But this is all worth it. Because the stuff mainstream brands use to keep their product from drying out—propylene glycol—is *antifreeze*. Yup. And it's known to cause brain, liver, and kidney abnormalities. Some effective natural brands to try: Crystal Essence, Soapwalla, Tom's of Maine. (Making the switch is easier if you keep your mainstream powerhouse deodorant in the medicine cabinet for special occasions.)

WORK STANDING UP

One day our grandkids will laugh at the fact that we sat at desks instead of standing, just as kids today are shocked by the fact that there was a time when no one wore seat belts and everyone smoked. We're built to be on two legs, not on our butts all day. Even in the best possible chair, sitting tightens up the hips and lower back and atrophies your walking muscles. Stand-up desks are the wave of the future. If you have the option to choose one (or rig one up) at your office, go for it.

MAKE A HEALTHY BED

Add an organic topper to your bed as a barrier against the chemicals used to make conventional mattresses, and when the time comes for a new mattress, look for one that's made of natural latex, cotton, or wool. Use unbleached cotton bedding, not synthetics (which are often treated with chemicals) and natural materials on the floor, like wool or sisal. And no electric blankets. Go old-school with a hot water bottle instead.

COLOR FOR MOOD MANIPULATION

Certain hues—in small or large doses—have a profound impact on the way you feel in your home. Whether you paint a wall, add a throw to your bed, or rethink the collection of objects on your kitchen windowsill, you can use color to support your spirit.

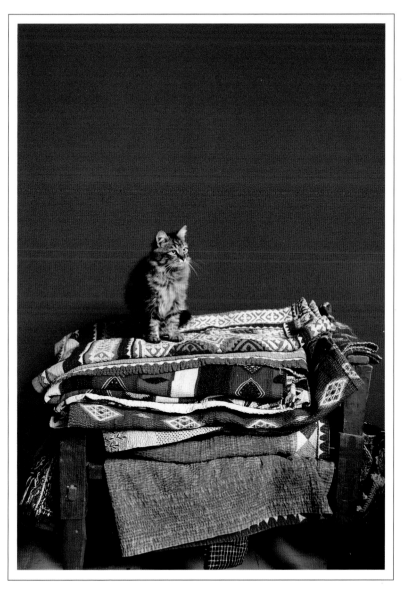

Red is energizing (though maybe not for this guy).

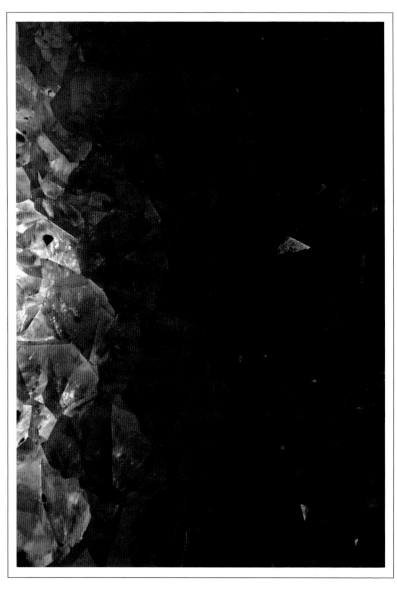

Lavender encourages contemplation.

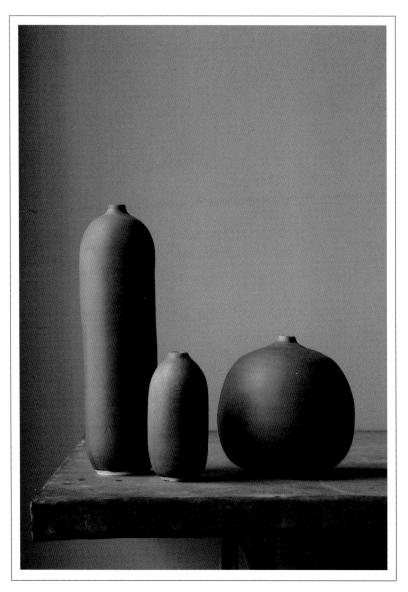

Blue brings calm.

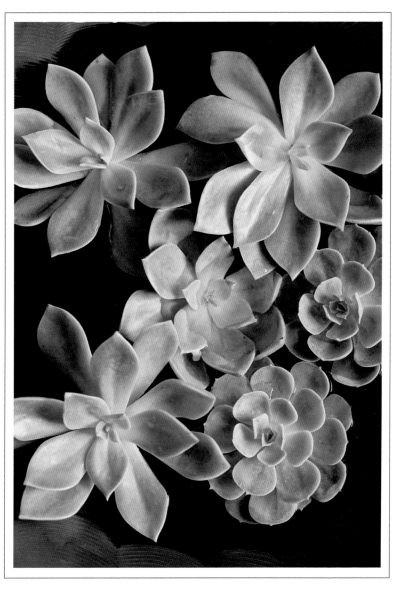

Light green can make you feel hopeful.

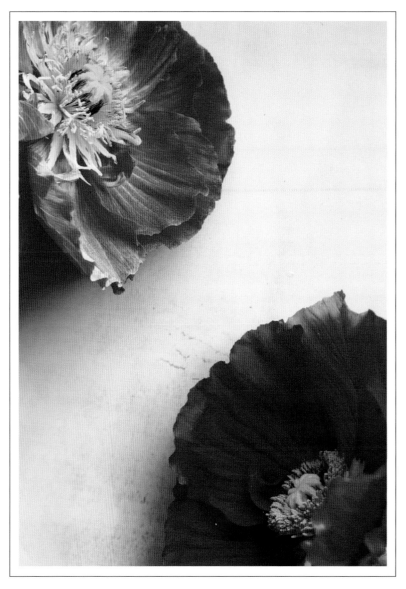

Orange makes you happy.

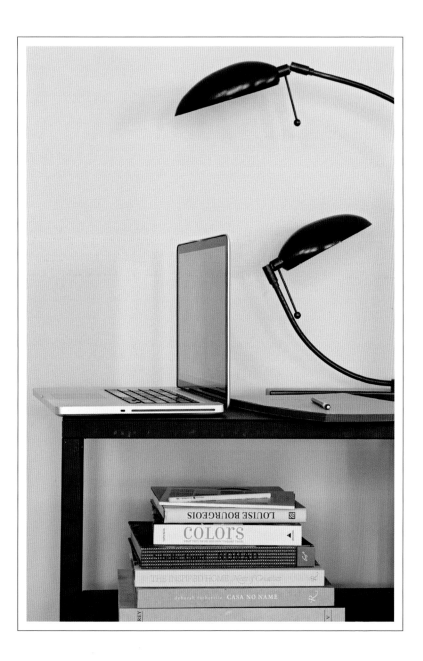

CLUTTER IS THE JUNK FOOD OF THE HOME

Clearing it out ungunks the gears and gets energy moving again. Your soul and brain feel better and function more smoothly in a place that's been purged of extraneous objects. So throw out junk; find a person (or an organization) to donate useful items to in an ongoing way; set up a system for organizing keepsakes; and—most important—buy less stuff.

SOOTHE YOUR SURROUNDINGS

Following a few basic tenets of feng shui in your home can improve your mental, physical, and spiritual well-being. Top of the list: Toss or fix broken objects—a stopped clock, a loose doorknob, a busted fan. These dead or weakened items are hard on the spirit of a room. Second, make rooms easy to move through—keep entryways clear (as in, don't crowd them with large furniture pieces). Third, introduce round shapes instead of sharp corners when you can. Think of a circular or oval coffee table, a round mirror. Curves are soothing; corners can feel aggressive. Fourth, add in something to energize a space. This could be touches of the color red (a powerful hue in feng shui); something that moves, like a mobile; or something that's alive—plants or pets. Try it. You'll feel it.

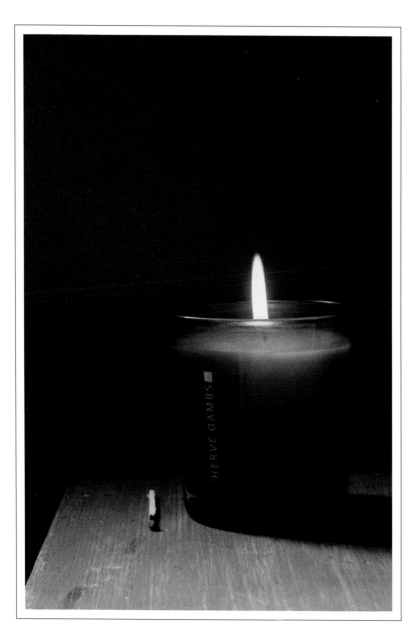

ACKNOWLEDGMENTS

Danielle Claro: Many thanks to Lia Ronnen and the wonderful team at Artisan; David Larabell, agent extraordinaire; Andrea Gentl and Marty Hyers, whose stunning photography goes beyond what I could have imagined; and Renata Di Biase, our beautiful and skilled yoga model. Sincere thanks to Liz Kiernan and Danny Maloney, two friends who gave endless creative input, from proposal to proofs; Alan Stein for his invaluable insight and wisdom; and Beth Kobliner for her friendship and faith in this project and all my projects. Thanks to Larry Smith for a great workshop and perpetual nudging, and to Stephanie Sisco for her crack organizational skills. Deep thanks (from the bottom of my feet) to Cyndi Lee, and all my wonderful teachers at Om and Now Yoga. Thanks to my parents and my four siblings, who infuse everything I write. And thanks last and most of all to my kids, Ian Reilly and Ruby Reilly, two amazing people who teach me more than I could ever teach them—in a book or otherwise.

Frank Lipman, M.D.: A big thanks to Danielle Claro, who conceived a beautiful vision and brought it to fruition. As always, I am indebted to my wonderful wife, Janice, and daughter, Alison, for their unwavering support. A huge shout-out to my staff at Eleven Eleven Wellness Center: Victoria Zodo, Anne Murray, Dr. Keren Day, Dr. Tina Discepola, Scott Berliner, Vanessa Echeverria, and Kate Horrigan. To my amazing team of Be Well Health Coaches: Kerry Bajaj, Jennifer Mielke, Katrine Van Wyk, Courtney Blatt, Jenny Sansouci, Laura Kraber, Jackie Damboragian, and Amanda Carney. Special thanks to my agent, Stephanie Tade, for making this happen. To Lindsey Clennell—yoga teacher, mentor, brother, and so much more—for keeping me mentally and physically grounded. To Jake Lief, Banks Gwaxula, and the rest of the Ubuntu Education Fund family, whose work continues to inspire me. And finally to my trusting patients, who constantly teach me and fuel my passion to create a healthier world.

ABOUT THE AUTHORS

FRANK LIPMAN, M.D., is a pioneer and global leader in the field of health and functional medicine. In 1992, he founded New York City's Eleven Eleven Wellness Center, where his brand of healing has helped thousands reclaim their zest for life, and in 2010 he developed Be Well by Dr. Frank Lipman, a line of cutting-edge health programs and supplements that recalibrate the body with healthy nutrients, vitamins, and minerals. A leading international speaker on wellness, he has been featured in *Vogue; Men's Journal; O, The Oprah Magazine*; and many other national magazines. This is his third book.

DANIELLE CLARO is a writer, editor, and longtime yogi who was founding editor in chief of the indie magazine *Breathe* and special projects director at *Domino* magazine. She's currently deputy editor of *Real Simple*.